Praise for *Get a Grip!*

"Amye Leong tells the story of her battle with arthritis with clarity. . . . This is inspirational reading for patients, for their physicians, and for anyone who knows someone with a chronic disease."

EDWARD HARRIS, JR., M.D., former president,
American College of Rheumatology
GEORGE DEFOREST BARNETT, Professor of Medicine,
Stanford University School of Medicine

"I laughed! I cried for joy and sadness! I clapped as I read Amye's story. She speaks with the authenticity of having 'been there' on the battlefield. You only make yourself worse if you try to run away from or fight chronic illness. Amye shows with integrity, honesty, courage, and humor how to live successfully with arthritis!"

KATHLEEN S. LEWIS, R.N., M.S., LPC, CMP,
medical psychotherapist and author of *Celebrate Life:
New Attitudes for Living with Chronic Illness*

"I have had the opportunity to know and observe Amye since my days at the National Arthritis Foundation, beginning in 1995. Amye was, and is, a truly positive force in the Arthritis Foundation. She was an eloquent spokesperson and conveyed hope by her messages, which connected with people with arthritis. She has had an even greater effect, by her examples, as a positive, charismatic, productive person with arthritis. She has expanded her reach to positively impact people with arthritis and lobby on their behalf worldwide, now as spokesperson for the Bone and Joint Decade effort. This book is her story, her insight, expressed openly and succinctly. It will provide guidance and hope to people with arthritis and their loved ones."

DOYT L. CONN, M.D., former senior vice president,
Medical Affairs, Arthritis Foundation; Professor of Medicine and
Director of Allergy, Immunology, and Rheumatology,
Emory School of Medicine

"Amye Leong's life is an inspiration to people affected by any chronic disorder and to the health professionals who care for them. Crippling arthritis washed away her childhood dream of living in France, but through her determination and, ironically, because of arthritis, she is now living that dream as official spokesperson for the United Nations/World Health Organization–endorsed Bone and Joint Decade. This book, Get a Grip!, chronicles her challenges and masterfully details the lessons she learned. It will help all arthritis sufferers not only live with the disease, but succeed in spite of it."

LARS LIDGREN, M.D., PH.D., Professor and chairman,
International Steering Committee, Bone and Joint Decade 2000–2010
chairman, Department of Orthopaedics, Lund University Hospital

"Amye's story is a 'must read' for anyone who has arthritis or cares about someone who does. Amye's journey from victim to accomplished advocate, public speaker, and businesswoman has served to inspire her countless friends at the Arthritis Foundation. Now this 'Arthritis Foundation treasure' is sharing her powerful story with all who feel challenged by chronic disease and want to reach within to find the resources necessary to take control, 'get a grip,' and begin to live their lives fully despite ever-continuing pain and disability."

DEBRA R. LAPPIN, J.D.,
former chair, Arthritis Foundation

GET A GRIP!

GET A GRIP!

A Take-Charge Approach
to Living with Arthritis

AMYE LEONG
WITH JOE LAYDEN

JEREMY P. TARCHER/PUTNAM

A MEMBER OF PENGUIN PUTNAM INC.

NEW YORK

Jeremy P. Tarcher/Putnam
a member of
Penguin Putnam Inc.
375 Hudson Street
New York, NY 10014

Library of Congress Cataloging-in-Publication Data

Leong, Amye.
Get a grip! : a take-charge approach to living
with arthritis/Amye Leong, with Joe Layden.
p.   cm.
ISBN 1-58542-148-0
1. Leong, Amye—Health.
2. Arthritis—Patients—United States—Biography.
I. Layden, Joseph, date.   II. Title.
RC933.L44   2002   2001058582
362.1'96722'0092—dc21
[B]

Printed in the United States of America
3   5   7   9   10   8   6   4   2

This book is printed on acid-free paper. ∞

BOOK DESIGN BY MEIGHAN CAVANAUGH

This book is dedicated to my mom and dad, Jeanne and Harvey Leong, whose consummate love, care, and support helped me heal, grow, and prosper. Although Dad passed away before seeing me realize my dream of thriving in Paris, I know he's watching out for me from Heaven and smiling.

This is for you, Dad and Mom!

ACKNOWLEDGMENTS

This book would not have been possible without that first conversation with Frank Coffey and George Alevizos on a Venice, California, balcony overlooking the blue Pacific. Thanks to Frank Weimann of Literary Group International for believing in our project and to Mark Meyerson, whose trusted legal eye and friendship opened new doors. And thanks to our editor at Penguin Putnam, Denise Silvestro, whose undying belief, guidance, expertise, and patience made this book a reality. For enthusiastic support and parting the waves for us, our thanks to publisher Joel Fotinos, and Joanne Kenny and Brian Underwood at Penguin Putnam.

Along this never-a-dull-moment journey, a boatload of family and friends helped me turn a problem into a challenge and then beaucoup opportunities. For the love that only family can bring, I thank my sister, Christine Leong Lynch; my niece, Amye Michelle Chow; and nephews, Nicholas David and Christopher Elliot Chow. For lifelong Chinese-style encouragement, I thank uncles and aunts, Gene and Laura Leong, Martha and Eugene Lowe, M.D., and Mabel and Joe Woo, M.D. For enduring love, understanding, and soulful support, I thank Robert Hutto, who has always believed in me, even when I didn't. And I thank my dearest friends who are family, my beloved "sistah" Sarah, Mikie, and Barton Richman for their deep, abiding love. For their universal humor, love, and unending capacity to keep me sane, I thank Daniel Patrick "beep-beep" Anderson, Ronski and Judy Norton, and Michael "go get 'em" Hakan. And I thank my gritty arthritis soul sisters whom I love to the core, Linda "Eggs" Wilson, Julia "Dolly" McClanahan, Janet "Cappuccino" Austin, and my yet-to-be-nicknamed sisters, Norine Walker and Edie Nixon. Arthritis brought us together, but deep love and sisterly confidence will keep us together even after we find a cure.

I thank the loving friends who made a difference in my arthritis and continue to enliven my life, Tina Goldfarb Moses, Mary Ellen Kullman Courtright, Sister Pam Flaherty, Jan Rasmussen, Brother Tom Juneman, Lee Miller, Gary Gee, Dick and Peggy Hays, Carol and Harry Saal, Woody Woodward, Jessica Saal, Joan Wong, Gordon "GP" Potter, and Judy Cohen of Medical Information Services.

Thanks to my Arthritis Foundation family, the Southern California and Northern California chapters, all of my friends at the National Office in Atlanta, Georgia, and the volunteer leadership. There could be no better second family. I thank Armin "Rick" Kuder, Esq., for his mentorship, support, and guidance. And to the young-adult arthritis groups around the United States that saw what we developed in California and took it upon themselves to grow a movement, making me feel like the mother of them all, I thank Cindy Chow, Kathy Neff, Mary O'Donnell, Kevin Purcell, and Vince Santos.

And to the team of rheumatologists and orthopaedic surgeons who rebuilt me year by year and taught me my biggest role in recovery is being their team partner, my appreciation and gratitude go to Louis Kramer, M.D., Gideon Darvish, M.D., Dan Wallace, M.D., Ken Nies, M.D., Elaine Lambert, M.D., Steve Schwartz, M.D., Larry Dorr, M.D., Charles Neer, M.D., Andrea Cracchiolo, M.D., Harvard Ellman, M.D., Roy Meals, M.D., and Chris Mow, M.D.

And finally, but most important, my sincere appreciation and thanks go to my book partner, Joe Layden, who heard my stories and turned them into pure literary art.

CONTENTS

Introduction

Nothing can prevent the birds of misfortune from flying about your head, but it is up to you whether they nest in your hair.

CHINESE PROVERB

Life is like an ice cream cone—you have to learn to lick it.

CHARLIE BROWN

The birds of misfortune swooped down upon me in a black swarm nearly three decades ago, during my freshman year at the University of California at Santa Barbara. It was then that I was first diagnosed with rheumatoid arthritis, a chronic, debilitating, incurable disease with an enormous capacity for inflicting pain and humiliation upon its unfortunate host. I'm not proud to say that my initial response to this development was a rather feeble stew of disbelief, self-pity, and surrender. But that's the way it happened. Today I've grown accustomed to shooing the birds away. If I haven't exactly learned how to lick life, I've at least learned how to put up a pretty good fight.

Get a Grip! is at once my story and my personal formula for coping successfully with this disease; it is the result of one woman's search for dignity and meaning in a life profoundly and perpetually affected by illness. Since 1984, I have endured sixteen arthritis-related surgeries, including twelve joint replacements. I have artificial elbows, artificial shoulders, artificial knees, artificial toes, and artificial knuckles. I've had reconstructive work on my hands and wrists. In my ongoing struggle to delay an inevitable cervical spine fusion, I've graduated from a ten-dollar neck brace to a four-hundred-dollar neck brace. In a very real sense, I am the Bionic Woman. Unfortunately, I don't move like the Bionic Woman. I have neither superhuman strength nor speed. And, since the prostheses that now encompass a large percentage of my body need periodic tune-ups and replacements, there is no end in sight. This battle will be waged until the day I die or a cure is found.

The point, however, is not simply that I have been pummeled by rheumatoid arthritis. I'm not looking for pity. My admittedly immodest goal in writing this book is to inspire and assist, to make the general public aware of the pervasiveness of this disease, and, especially, to let other people with arthritis know that even in the most extreme cases—and it can be among the most cruel of illnesses—there is cause for hope. Lots of it!

As a past chair of the American Juvenile Arthritis Organization, a member of the Advisory Council of the National Institute of Arthritis and Musculoskeletal and Skin Diseases, and spokesperson for the Bone and Joint Decade, I have been fortunate to work with many of America's leading health-care professionals. Through my work as a motivational speaker and as a member of the Board of Directors of the Arthritis Foundation, I've had the opportunity to share my views and experiences with scientists, physicians, physical therapists, occupational therapists, corporate leaders, legislators, and lobbyists. Most of them have said to me, individually or in presentations, "Amye, I don't know that I've ever seen a case of rheumatoid arthritis as severe as yours. I don't know anyone who has been through quite as much." To which I usually reply, "Well, thank you very much. Now . . . what can we do to reduce the possibility of anyone else ever going through the same thing in the future? And what can we do to help the millions of people who are currently struggling to cope with this disease?"

This book, I hope, represents part of the answer. I can tell you from personal experience that growing up with arthritis is extraordinarily challenging. Most people don't realize that arthritis, at its worst, can rob you of your will to live. I have reached that point myself, and as a peer counselor I've had young people call me on the phone, in tears, and tell me that the gun was sitting next to them, and they were willing to use it. That's another misconception about arthritis—that it is exclusively a disease of the elderly. Not true. In fact, according to the National Bureau of Health Statistics, there are more than eight million people under the age of forty-five in the United States who suffer from some form of debilitating arthritis. That's an awful lot of people—greater than the number of people who have chronic bronchitis.

I've been fortunate. I hit rock bottom and somehow, with the grace of God, and the unwavering support of friends and family, propelled myself back up. The story of that journey, I have been told, is something that people around the country have wanted to hear . . . have *needed* to hear, because even if they haven't experienced the severity of the disease that I have, they've certainly experienced some of the emotional garbage that goes along with it. If this book can give readers a glimmer of hope—if it can help them realize that they are not alone, and provide them with the impetus to take control of their lives and their treatment—then I will have succeeded.

A more ambitious goal is to change public perception. There are 43 million people in the United States with arthritis, and the Centers for Disease Control expects that figure to escalate at an astonishing pace as our population continues to age. Within twenty years, the number of people afflicted with arthritis will be approximately 60 million! By any reasonable definition, that must be considered an epidemic. And the World Health Organization has confirmed that rheumatoid arthritis, within a decade after onset, leads to work disability in as many as 59 percent of those of us affected. And yet, arthritis remains a largely misunderstood ailment, its victims a greatly underserved community. I want to educate people about the severity and seriousness of this disease; I want to sensitize them. Most important of all, I want to call them to action.

There is a level of education I would like to address in this book, beginning with an explanation of terms. When most people talk about arthritis, they are referring to the type of arthritis we may all get, someday, provided we are fortunate enough to live that long. This is known as osteoarthritis, which is caused by joint deterioration brought on by old age or genetic weakness, or trauma—athletic injuries, for example. Osteoarthritis can be a gnawing nuisance or cause extreme pain; there's no doubt about that. And there is no cure yet. But there are more than a hundred other types of arthritis, such as rheumatoid arthritis, that are far more serious and that can indeed lead to an early death. Without appropriate care you can die from lupus or from scleroderma. You can have such severe complications from rheumatoid arthritis that you develop potentially dangerous heart and respiratory problems. When we talk about arthritis we are not simply talking about a joint problem. We are not merely talking about someone who has trouble getting up and down the stairs. We're talking about systemic problems that have life-threatening repercussions.

I also want people to understand the emotional consequences of living with a so-called "hidden disability." For many people with arthritis, that is the most debilitating and challenging aspect of arthritis. To the untrained eye, there are many days when it would be hard to tell that I have rheumatoid arthritis. When I was hospitalized or confined to a wheelchair or forced to use platform crutches, then it was obvious. The absence of those things, however, does not mean the pain has disappeared. I can look across a room—any room—and tell you exactly who has arthritis, just by watching their movements. How they walk. How they move their body when they sit down. How they turn their head, as if they have an acute stiff neck. It's the way someone gets out of a chair. It's the way someone doesn't rush to a door to get through it when it's shutting, because they simply can't, because it hurts too much.

I see these things—I *feel* them—because I am a twenty-five-year veteran of this war. The casual observer hasn't a clue. Perception, in fact, is among the biggest challenges that anyone with arthritis faces. If you were to watch me get out of my car after parking in a space designated for disabled drivers, you'd likely give me a stern look and perhaps even a reprimand: "Hey, that's for a handicapped person, and you're not handicapped!" I would respond by saying, "I have arthritis." And you'd probably say in disbelief, "Yeah, right!"

Arthritis pain can be excruciating. It can cut the heart out of your self-esteem. But even more exhausting is the relentless struggle of having to explain to others why you don't fit into their image of arthritis.

You won't hear me preach in this book. Instead, I hope, the various themes unfold naturally, through the telling of my story. It is not merely a story of pain and suffering, but of love, friendship, and family. It is, ultimately, a triumphant story, not because I have been cured—for now, that remains an impossibility—but because I am overcoming this disease in my own mind. I am fighting it with all my emotional, mental, spiritual, and attitudinal strength. If there is one message I want to share with you, the reader, it is this: Arthritis is not an end point. You may feel that you have no control over your life, that you have, in fact, been given a death sentence (or, at least, a sentence of life without parole). But there are always options.

As I travel around the world, speaking to audiences about arthritis, I hear the same questions over and over: "How do you stay so positive?" "How did you get out of that wheelchair and become able to move so well now?" "How do you stay focused?" Each encounter with the surgeon's knife is a test, each flare a challenge. I am in this for the long haul, so I must be resilient, and the key to resilience is laughter. Humor is an important part of my life. I'm not talking about cynicism, because I think cynicism can be deadly; it's anger pushed inside, and it solves nothing. When I sense the cynic in me bubbling to the surface, I'll drive to the beach, park my car, and try to shout over the din of the breaking waves. I will curse arthritis and all it has done to me: ravaged my body, stolen my independence, stripped me of the ability to have children. Then, when my throat is raw and the hateful words stop coming, I get back in the car and drive home, and work on my action plan.

Most of the time, though, I'm able to laugh at myself and appreciate the circumstances that have led me to this place. Pain and humor aren't so far apart on the emotional scale, I've discovered, and laughter truly is the best medicine. Even in a life punctuated by tremendous challenge, there is so much to cherish and there are so many positive choices to be made. I think you'll agree.

A Loss of Dignity

The saddest moment—the scariest moment—came not in a surgical suite or a doctor's office but in a beautiful waterfront apartment, in the cool blackness of night.

I was in my twenties at the time and living in Marina del Rey, California. For more than a decade I had waged a halfhearted battle with rheumatoid arthritis, rarely giving the disease its due, and almost never acknowledging its overwhelming presence in my life. My family was aware of my condition, of course, as were a few close friends. In general, though, I downplayed its significance, denied its increasingly obvious influence on my mind and body. Rheumatoid arthritis is a long-term, degenerative disease with a ferocious, indiscriminate appetite, as well as an enormous capacity to inflict pain on its host. Unfortunately, it has a bit of an image problem.

Like most people, I had labored under the mistaken impression that arthritis afflicted only the elderly. Even then, as my life and career continued to spiral downward due to massive physical pain, I was reluctant to admit the simple truth: that I was one of the eight million young adults in the United States who suffered from this ailment. That I would one day become fodder for medical texts—a living, breathing example of rheumatoid arthritis at its most devastating was inconceivable.

Even as my health deteriorated, I stubbornly, enthusiastically embraced a philosophy of denial, in large part because I feared the consequences of going public. I had a promising career as a human resources manager with GTE, a vibrant, growing company that seemed to think quite highly of my abilities, and I was reluctant to reveal anything that might put my professional future at risk. GTE was as progressive as any company around, but this was in the 1980s, and the corporate environment at the time was much different than it is today, especially for women. There were very few young people in executive positions, and those who had risen quickly were smart, attractive, and very healthy-looking. You had to be blind not to pick up on that, and I wasn't blind. I decided early in my tenure that I would project an image of confidence, vitality, and health, even if it wasn't entirely accurate.

When I had first joined GTE a few years earlier, straight out of an MBA program at Purdue University, my arthritis was manageable; it did not affect my ability to work. There had been flares in the past, some so severe that they required hospitalization, but I never volunteered that information. It just wasn't relevant. To me they were a distant memory, remnants of another life. I was young and naive and thought, somehow, that perhaps I had "beaten" the disease. But I was wrong. You can't beat arthritis. Since there is no cure, the best you can hope for is a stalemate. The struggle is constant, isolating, enduring.

For a while I worked with feverish intensity, just like anyone else with serious aspirations. I was promoted into a supervisory position. I enjoyed the camaraderie, the competition, the first heady whiff of power. I enjoyed the money I was making.

I was putting in sixty-five-hour workweeks, basically living at the office, and the predictable result of this schedule was an eroding of my social life; even worse, my body was beginning to crumble beneath the weight of so much stress. At the time it seemed as though the crisis arrived almost without warning, although in retrospect I realize that wasn't the case at all. There was a steadiness to the progression of the disease, a boldness that made it nearly impossible to ignore. I just wasn't paying attention. Until, finally, I had no choice.

Each morning it took me a little longer to get going. The smallest tasks became tremendous chores. Merely getting dressed, something as simple as putting on a pair of slacks, required extraordinary effort. My knuckles were so swollen that I couldn't grasp the zipper and pull it up. My wrists and elbows were so inflamed that it was a struggle just to lift a toothbrush to my mouth. In the final weeks, as I approached bottom, I developed an exhausting, insane routine. I'd rise at four in the morning after a few hours of fitful sleep, pop a few pain pills, reset the alarm, and close my eyes for thirty minutes. By the time the alarm went off again, the medication would have kicked in enough to dull the stabbing pain, and I'd be able to begin the process of getting ready for another day. I'd stand up, slowly walk to the bathroom, turn on the shower, and start working out the kinks. I felt like I was encased in cement, unable to move at all. After about forty-five minutes in the shower, the next tier of pain was dulled enough and I would start to come to life. Only then did I have relief enough to get dressed, put on some makeup, and drive myself to work.

With each successive day the duration of my "morning stiffness," as it is so euphemistically called, increased. Eventually I found myself arriving at the office at ten A.M., ten-thirty, eleven. I was still getting up before dawn, but that wasn't enough. The act of preparing for work now consumed nearly as much time as the workday itself. As a manager I was not required to punch a clock. It didn't matter when I came to work or how many hours I put in. As long as I did the job, my boss was satisfied. So I'd stay at the office until seven or eight in the evening, go home, sleep for a few hours, and then do it all over again.

As my condition worsened, I confided in my supervisor. I really had no other choice—it was obvious that I was in deep trouble. I was shuffling around the office like an old woman, my eyes fixed on the floor so that I wouldn't trip, and so that no one could see the pain on my face. But I couldn't hide it. I'm five feet, two inches tall and I've never weighed more than 105 pounds. Now, though, I had eroded to an anorexic eighty pounds.

In my last few days at GTE I would call in and say, "I'm having a tough time today. If I can come in, I'll come in. But if I can't, I can't. Is that all right?" My boss was very sympathetic, very accommodating. "Take whatever time you need," he said. "Just let us know if there's anything we can do."

Of course, I still didn't want to admit defeat. As a self-sufficient woman I was loath to give anyone the impression that I needed help. I was too young to be moving around as if every step was going to be the last, especially in a professional environment where competition among peers was critical. My office was typical of corporate life in the 1980s. It was not the touchy-feely, team-building atmosphere of the '90s. Everybody was trying to get ahead, myself included. There was nothing evil about it. That's just the way it was. I was fortunate to have a trusting relationship with my boss, but I did not have that type of relationship with all my peers. Sometimes I'd walk into the office very slowly, and very late, and feel as though everyone was staring at me. It was hard not to be stung by the sarcasm when a co-worker said, "Gee, Amye, nice to see you this morning," or "Well, look who's here. Slumming today, Amye?" I was well aware that I could not project an image of helplessness, of sickness, of anything other than . . . *I'm in control. I'm in command.*

One of the most challenging and depressing characteristics of rheumatoid arthritis is that the severity of the disease is not always apparent. It can be quite puzzling not only to the person affected but also to those who see her on a regular basis. After all, I looked tired, drawn. But I wasn't in a cast. I wasn't using crutches or a wheelchair. There was nothing that visibly defined my illness. Even my boss had trouble understanding it. His intentions were good—his heart was in the right place—but I could tell he just didn't get it. And who could blame him? I'd be functional one day, sick the next. I'd come in later and later. When I finally told him what was happening, I could see a flicker of doubt and confusion in his eyes: *She's too young to have arthritis. What's going on?*

"I don't fully understand it myself," I told him. "Please, just work with me on it."

In hindsight, I realize I made the deliberate choice *not* to tell my boss about my condition for fear of retribution, disbelief, or simply being treated *differently.* Arthritis had never deeply affected the nature or quality of my work until then. But when it finally did, I had no choice but to reveal the nature of my illness—and what a relief that turned out to be! Sharing some of the details of your illness, especially with those who have an impact on your life (such as your family, friends, and employer), represents a major step toward asking for help and building support. And remember—the Americans with Disabilities Act guarantees a legal safety net for the fear of retribution that plagued my silence.

Not long after I told my boss about my arthritis, I conceded that I couldn't keep up with the pace any longer. As much as I hated to admit it, my body was giving out on me, and I needed to take an extended leave of absence from work.

Depression is common among the chronically ill, and I certainly fell into that category. Confined to my apartment, lonely, unable to work, enveloped in pain, I experienced a sadness unlike anything I'd ever known. Here I was in a gorgeous, expensive apartment in Marina del Rey—the prime place to be when you're young and single in southern California—but when I looked out the window I didn't see the beautiful boats or the sun shining or the people running around in shorts and bathing suits. All I could see was pain. All I could see was darkness. I shuffled from room to room, trying to keep my bathrobe from sliding off my shoulders, because I knew I did not have the strength to put it back on. I avoided mirrors because I hated what I saw. Gone was the bright-eyed high-school homecoming queen. In her place was someone unrecognizable—a pathetic, incongruous creature with a face bloated by massive doses of prednisone teetering atop the emaciated frame of a famine victim. In sum, I looked like a lollipop.

The pain at that time was excruciating. Virtually all my major weight-bearing joints—knees, ankles, feet, shoulders, hands—were inflamed. As bone rubbed against bone, I sometimes nearly passed out from the pain. It felt as if someone had taken knives and stuck them into my joints and left them there. And every time I moved, the blades moved. It was a sharp, piercing, "I can't think straight" kind of pain. Imagine lifting your arm and resting your hand on a table. It seems so innocuous to me now. Then it was pure agony. I was, quite literally, crippled. Even the little circuit I had developed—from chair to bed to bathroom—became almost unmanageable.

One evening in March, I sat for hours in the dark, crying, on the verge of panic. I tried to calm myself: *You'll get through this, Amye. You just need to get some sleep.* But I couldn't sleep, even though persistent, intense pain is exhausting. It's as if someone is bombarding you with the worst music imaginable, so loud that you can't think or concentrate on anything else. Lying in bed, in a fetal position, surrounded by pillows, I would doze off for ten or fifteen minutes, only to be awakened by a shot of stabbing pain. For hours I hung on the ragged edge of consciousness, lost in a fog of pain and painkillers.

It went on like that all night. Finally, around two-thirty in the morning, the crisis really hit. I woke to the realization that I needed to go to the bathroom and tried to raise myself off the bed . . . but

I couldn't. I was helpless. Despite all I had been through—despite the precipitous decline in my physical state—this came as something of a shock. Imagine what it takes to get out of bed, how easy and simple it seems. *Sit up. Slide your legs over the edge. Stand up. Walk.* Suddenly, I could do none of those things. The pain in my arms and shoulders was so severe that I could not lift myself off the bed. I was too weak. I had to find another way.

I turned on my right hip and tried to shift all of my weight to my right buttock. Then I began to sway back and forth, very slowly at first, then faster. Eventually, after about twenty minutes, I used my momentum to bring myself up into a sitting position. Unfortunately, that simple act took all of my strength. I was utterly spent. I wanted to put my feet on the floor and walk to the bathroom, but I couldn't. It was an approach-avoidance situation. It's hard to do something when you know that the more you try to do it, the worse the pain is going to be. It's like one of those adventure stories in which the crocodile has a gleaming jewel resting in its open mouth. You want the jewel, and it's tempting to reach down and try to grab it. But you know the beast is going to snap its jaws shut and cut off your arm if you try. So it's not worth the risk.

Sitting there in bed, all alone, unable to control or even recognize my own body, I began to shake. I'd never been so frightened in my entire life.

It's difficult to explain what goes through your mind in a situation like that. Suddenly, nothing seems to matter. I didn't think about calling out for help. All I wanted to do was go to the bathroom. Was that such an unreasonable request? I just wanted to use the bathroom like a normal human being, something that was so rote and so easy to do . . . something I'd been doing without effort or thought since I was a toddler. It was at precisely that moment, when my sense of dignity was swept away, that I was completely consumed by this disease. And it was terrifying. I felt as though I had lost my life. I felt less than human. I felt like I was just some . . .

thing . . . that needed to use the toilet. I didn't have a brain, I didn't have wants, and I didn't have needs. I didn't have a vision of what my life was all about. None of that made sense anymore. None of it mattered. My entire existence was distilled into this elemental act— a simple, basic bodily function. An animalistic function.

When I realized that I couldn't perform this function in the customary manner, in the way society deems appropriate, I crumbled. I became a child again. And like any child in the throes of a crisis, I reached out for my mommy and daddy.

I could have called one of my neighbors. I could have called a girlfriend. I could have dialed 911 and shouted, "Help! I can't go to the bathroom!" But I chose to call my parents who lived one hundred fifty miles away, in Bakersfield. I reached for the phone, which was next to my bed, and began to dial.

My father answered. "Hello."

"Dad . . . " I couldn't vocalize much more than that at first. I was in too much pain. I was too scared.

"Amye," he said. "What's wrong?"

He knew right away it was me, even though my voice was barely audible, my words almost unintelligible. And he knew something was terribly wrong. There was a desperation that I couldn't hide, didn't want to hide. My father and I were extraordinarily close. He had a way of knowing when I was in trouble, when I was having a bad day. It wasn't unusual for him to call and say, "Are you all right today, Amye? I just had a feeling, and I wanted to make sure." He'd ask me if I was eating properly, if I was taking my medication. In recent months the calls had been less frequent because he knew that I was trying to take care of myself, and at some point a parent has to respect the wishes of an adult child. But he never stopped worrying.

Through tears I choked out, "I have to go to the bathroom, Dad. And I can't move."

There was a pause.

"Well, Amye, just wet the bed. I'll be down to your place in a couple of hours."

As soon as he said those words, the adult in me nudged the child aside. *How stupid is it that you called your father to tell him you couldn't go to the bathroom? You need professional help, kid. You don't need your father.* That's part of the recovery process: knowing when to admit that you need help—real help. The very first step to reclaiming control over your life—and your disease—is becoming aware of what you need. This awareness comes on like a lightbulb.

Hearing him actually say "wet the bed" was an awakening. It sounded so silly and facetious, but it really wasn't funny at all. *Yeah, right, Dad. Just wet the bed. I'm so embarrassed.* Sorry, I wasn't ready to accept that.

"You know what, Dad?" I said. "This is ridiculous. Don't drive the three hours all the way down here. I'll be all right."

"What are you going to do?"

"I'll call Tina. She'll come over and help."

Tina Goldfarb was a physical therapist who worked for Daniel Freeman Memorial Hospital. She was also a good friend who lived only a short distance away.

After a while, my father relented. "Okay," he said. "But after she gets there, please call me back."

"I will."

"I love you, Amye."

"I love you too, Dad."

When it came to handling difficult situations, Tina was a pro. We had met only a few months earlier, at a seminar on arthritis. By chance we sat next to each other. Since we were both attending the conference alone, we ended up having lunch together. The conversation was light, comfortable. We quickly became friends. I valued her companionship and trusted her judgment. Looking back on it, our meeting seems to have been more than mere coincidence. But then, I've been fortunate in that regard. Throughout my life the appropriate resources have been available when I needed them most, like flowers blooming on a dark and dismal day.

I dialed Tina's number. When she answered, I began crying again. I explained the situation.

"Hang on," she said. "It'll take me about an hour, but I'll be there for you."

"Tina . . . I can't wait an hour."

She chuckled. "Look, Amye, it's all right. Just let it go."

There it was again. Everyone wanted me to pee in my pants. Didn't they understand how humiliating it was? How disgusting? Unfortunately, there really was no other option. I hung up the phone and settled back onto the pillows to wait for my friend. After a while my muscles relaxed, and nature, in all its humbling glory, took its course. At nearly thirty years of age, with tears streaming down my cheeks, I wet the bed.

2

Arthritis? That's for Old People

Growing up in Bakersfield, California, in the 1960s was all about fun. My family had a big old house in the middle of town—a wonderful, traditional house with a sprawling red porch overlooking a yard dotted with trees. I spent a lot of time on that porch, just hanging out, reading, doing puzzles, watching the world drift by at a leisurely pace, a pace that often seemed a bit too slow for me. You see, I was a very active kid. And kind of an odd kid, too, I guess. Other kids liked candy and soda and popcorn—junk like that. I liked olives. One of my favorite things to do was to put pitted olives on my fingertips and try to climb my favorite tree. This was a Herculean feat, trying to scurry up a tree using only my legs and the palms of my hands, but I always managed to do it without getting hurt or, worse, crushing my precious olives. I was a little monkey, always climbing fences, trees, anything that looked inviting. I never sensed danger in these activities, just fun and adventure.

I was a healthy kid growing up in a healthy home. Aside from getting tossed around once in a while by my older sister, J (short for Jay-Jay, which means "big sister" in Chinese, even though her real name is Christine), I never experienced any bumps or bruises. I was almost never sick. In fact, my entire family was healthy. And when I talk about family, I'm not just talking about Mom and Dad and Sis. As is often the case in Chinese-American families, I was raised in close proximity to numerous aunts and uncles and cousins and grandparents. We were a very close family. Interestingly, there is no history of arthritis whatsoever among any of my blood relatives. That doesn't necessarily mean anything, because even today we aren't sure whether a specific genetic component will inevitably lead to the disease. I have rheumatoid arthritis, but there is no certainty that my offspring would have it. Modern research seems to indicate, however, that there is a predisposition; unfortunately, that predisposition remains largely a mystery. Moreover, even after someone is diagnosed, we don't know whether the disease will be fast-acting or not; whether it will be severe or mild. We just don't know.

After I was diagnosed with arthritis, I spent a lot of time in medical libraries researching the disease. Eventually I found a link between rheumatoid arthritis and a skin condition called psoriasis that had long affected my mother, Jeanne. We now know that psoriasis, like rheumatoid arthritis, is a disease of the immune system. In essence, the two are cousins—distant cousins, perhaps, but relatives nonetheless. I don't remember Mom complaining about it much, but I do recall her scratching her legs a lot. Psoriasis can be very bad, with open sores that fail to heal properly and an incessant itching that can drive the patient practically mad. Mom's case was never like that. She had the typical type of psoriasis you might get in a place like Bakersfield, where the air is dry and the summertime temperature routinely soars into the hundreds. The climate is tough on dry skin, and for the longest time that's all we thought it was with Mom—an environmental condition. She rarely talked about her "itchy legs," and she was not inclined to visit doctors, even though my uncle Eugene, her brother, was an internist! To Mom, it was just dry skin . . . a part of life. Could Mom's psoriasis have been an indicator that I would eventually have rheumatoid arthritis? Maybe, maybe not. As I said, with arthritis we just don't know.

My dad, Harvey Leong, was the owner of a grocery store in town, the kind of place where everyone was on a first-name basis and customers could get almost anything they needed—from candy to thick deli sandwiches to household cleaners. I loved the weekends because I got to spend time with my dad, helping out in the store. I wasn't always the best assistant, though. People would stop by and talk, and I would reward their kindness and friendship by giving away samples of the candy. My dad often had to remind me that I was supposed to collect a dime for every piece of candy I handed out. The other neat thing was lunchtime, when we'd sit together in a small kitchen at the back of the store.

"Go pick out something for lunch," Dad would say.

"Like what?"

Invariably, he'd smile and add, "Anything you want."

What a great opportunity that was for a little girl. I tasted all kinds of exotic foods, things I might otherwise never have sampled. Sometimes I'd put together weird combinations, but my dad never rebuked me or made fun of my choices. I became very open to experimentation and problem-solving, concepts that have served me well in my battle with arthritis. I think it's fair to say that those early days were important preparation for meeting the challenges I face today. People often tell me that I seem flexible. I can change, adapt, move on. The truth is, adaptability is not just an asset when you have a progressive, incurable disease—it's a requirement. When you're dealing with a condition that is causing you immense pain on a daily basis, a condition that can flare up at any time and thus make it impossible for you to go on with your scheduled activities, you have to learn to be adaptable.

Think about when you were a child and you asked your parents for something you really wanted. If their response was "No!" did that stop you? Probably not. If you were like me, you figured out how to get around the word "no" by using your childlike creativity. Either adjust or be unhappy with the finality of "no."

In my ancestors' language, the Chinese word for "problem" is the same as the word for "opportunity." Coincidence? Not really. When you perceive a difficult situation as a problem, the walls seem so much higher to climb. But when you perceive the same difficult situation as an opportunity to learn about yourself and the world around you, options can open like floodgates. Perception makes all the difference in your strategy. In the peer counseling I provide, I've talked to a lot of people who labor under the misconception that rigidity is somehow an attribute. Well, at first rigidity might seem like a good idea because it implies strength of character and keeps you focused on the task at hand, which is fighting the disease. But when you're dealing with an illness that has so many ups and downs, whose course is so unpredictable, you have to develop a certain elasticity to cope with it. You want to bend, but not break.

It's strange how the simplest of things can add up to something important. I look back at my childhood, and I remember those days at the store with my dad . . . I remember climbing trees without using my fingertips . . . and I realize that something in those activities served a greater purpose. It helped make me the person I am today: a survivor.

In childhood I also learned the rudiments of advocacy. I was the first female president of my elementary school. Being president meant not only that I had to get my homework done every night, but also that I had to represent my classmates at PTA meetings and other administrative functions. Today I give more than one hundred speeches each year, and I'm quite comfortable with that type of interaction, but as a child, the very thought of standing in front of an audience and opening my mouth seemed daunting. The first time I was asked to speak in public was on a "teacher day," when kids got the day off while the faculty endured a full day of training sessions. All my friends were out playing and having fun, but I was in the largest auditorium in Bakersfield, giving a speech to several hundred teachers, administrators, and parents on the subject of "student needs." I remember pacing around backstage, feeling like I was going to faint or throw up. I was so nervous that I almost had to be pushed out to the podium. The lights blinded me, and my pretty little dress became drenched with sweat. Somehow, though, I got through it. I rambled on about what it was like to be an elementary student in Bakersfield, and how the teachers didn't really listen to the students. Already I was an advocate, although I didn't know it at the time.

Much later, during my senior year in high school, I was selected as the first student representative to the California Board of Education. The board was composed of politicians who met three or four times a year in Sacramento or Los Angeles to discuss the state of education in California and determine policy direction. Never before had there been student representation at these meetings, so I was pretty excited about taking part. I quickly learned, however, that when you're the "first" at anything, you spend a lot of your time breaking down barriers.

At my very first meeting I was astounded to see these people, these supposedly important and responsible adults, acting so nonchalant about such vital work—one man was even filing his fingernails during the meeting!—and they all treated me with such indifference. I really wanted to contribute; I wanted to understand the essence of what these meetings were about, and what these people were all about, but no one came over to say "Hi, welcome aboard" or anything like that. I had to go up to them and introduce myself, almost force them into a conversation.

I felt like I was trying to break a brick wall with my fingers. No one wanted to listen to me. The experience taught me an important lesson: When you're the first at something, don't expect an audience, but don't let that stop you. If something is important to you, and you have a passion for it, then be proactive. Don't assume that the issue is just as important to others. Take action, and your energy becomes a driving force that will make others take notice. But be passionate, take the initiative in your life's journey (you have my permission!), and especially in your medical care.

Some lessons were learned in a more traditional manner, like the time I tried my first cigarette. I was twelve years old, and at that age, of course, smoking seems like a pretty cool activity. (Remember, this was especially true in the 1960s and 1970s, before the Surgeon General's Office issued its blanket warning about the dangers of cigarette smoking.) My mother was working in a bank at the time, so my sister and I both had chores to complete as soon as we arrived home from school. We were expected to do our homework, clean up the house, set the table for dinner, even get dinner started. One day my girlfriend and I found a pack of my dad's cigarettes in the den, and we decided to go out in the backyard and light up. We shared a few lung-searing drags on a single cigarette, hated it, and went back inside. It really was a wretched experience, but somehow it made us feel just a bit more grown-up, which was, after all, the whole point.

Apparently, though, we weren't quite as smart as we thought, because that night I paid a price for my behavior. I didn't suspect anything at first. We had a nice family dinner, discussed the day's events, and then my sister and I did the dishes, just as we always did. Afterward, as I was walking down the hallway toward my bedroom, I heard Dad call out, "Amye, could you come here a minute? I'd like a word with you."

My heart fluttered. There was something in his tone that was different, something that told me, immediately, *You're in trouble, girl.*

I turned around and walked into the den, where my dad was waiting.

"Yeah, Dad?"

He rubbed his chin, as if gathering his thoughts.

"I hear you like to smoke," he said.

I froze in my tracks, unable to respond or even move. I was busted! Nevertheless, I resorted to that tried-and-true childhood defense: complete ignorance.

"What do you mean?"

He shook his head. "Come on, Amye. I hear you and Phyllis were out in the backyard this afternoon smoking my cigarettes. Well, if you like it that much, why don't you just smoke right here in the house?"

He reached into the breast pocket of his shirt and pulled out a fresh pack of Marlboros. I couldn't believe this was happening!

"Here," he said, fingering a fresh cigarette. "Have one of mine."

I had no idea how he had found out, but what was happening now was too weird for words—smoking with my father? Come on!

"Uhhhhh . . . that's okay, Dad," I stammered. "I'd rather not."

But Dad was not so easily dissuaded. He had a plan in mind, and he was going to see it through. "Amye," he said, "I want you to smoke this cigarette . . . now!"

He pulled out a lighter, gave it a flick, and soon the tip of the cigarette was glowing. I reluctantly, nervously, took it from his hands and placed it between my lips. Having no idea how to smoke a cigarette, I inhaled deeply and immediately began coughing in huge, dry spasms. My eyes turned red, my throat burned, my head began to spin. Sputtering, wheezing, I tried to give the cigarette back to my father, but he held up a hand and said, "Nope. Finish it. You want to smoke so much . . . go ahead and smoke."

My dad, who was ordinarily a very gentle man, proceeded to stand there as his daughter burned through an entire cigarette. He watched as I turned green and practically keeled over with nausea.

Afterward, he snuffed out the butt and sent me to my room. No further admonishment was necessary. To this day I can't even stand the smell of cigarette smoke; I get queasy just being the same room with someone who smokes—it had that great an impact on me. The irony, of course, is that my dad was a smoker (he has long since kicked the habit, by the way—been clean for more than twenty years). But he didn't want his daughter to smoke. It was a painful lesson, but it was also a profound expression of love, because it had a tremendous impact on me. I had thought smoking was cool, but smoking made me sick. After that, I never again wanted to do anything that could compromise my health or fitness.

As a child I was in perpetual motion. I loved to swim, so much that my parents used to call me "Esther Williams." I didn't know whom they were talking about, but I later found out Esther Williams was a great competitive swimmer who went on to appear in a string of movies in the 1950s. That seemed appropriate, since I could spend hours in the pool without getting tired. On land I was like a jackrabbit, always winning ribbons at local track competitions. I played tennis, too, thanks to the efforts of my uncle Gene, an accomplished player and a good teacher as well. This was before the advent of Title IX, so there weren't as many opportunities for girls to compete in high-school sports, but I took advantage of every opportunity there was. I loved competition. I loved the feeling of movement. I loved the energy! It never occurred to me then that it would all be taken away, that I would be relegated to the role of permanent spectator at an age when most people are still learning how to play the game.

As everyone knows, high school can be a harsh and cliquish world. I was one of the fortunate ones. I hung around with a good group of kids, had a lot of friends, never felt ostracized.

We weren't rich kids, just solidly middle class. We did our homework, played sports, and prepared for the next inevitable stage of our lives: college. But there's no denying that we were, like most kids, somewhat superficial. Adolescence in general, and high school in particular, is primarily about body image. What you wear and how you look matter every bit as much as who you are on the inside. That's unfair, of course, but it's an immutable fact of teenage life. My friends and I were extremely conscious of how we dressed, how we looked.

The attention I received in those days only made it harder for me to cope with the trauma of rheumatoid arthritis, so closely was my identity tied to my appearance. It was common then for girls to wear tights under short skirts—you know, the way Marcia dressed on *The Brady Bunch*. One day in my sophomore year I was walking across campus with a friend when a bunch of senior boys began whistling and yelling.

"Nice legs!" one of them said.

My girlfriend whirled around toward the group and hissed, "That's pretty stupid!"

The boy shook his head. "Not you," he shouted. Then he pointed at me. "Her!"

I have to admit, for a fifteen-year-old girl, that's a pretty flattering experience, and I took pride in it. I'd never actually had anyone whistle at me before . . . and a senior, to boot? That was all I needed. I had arrived! Please don't misunderstand me—I don't mean this in a boastful way. Teenagers are shallow, it's part of where they are in their lives, and I was no different. When you're in high school, there is nothing, and I mean nothing, more important than being popular. As we mature, we understand how silly this is. Part of being an adult, a valuable and thoughtful member of society, is understanding that you must get past appearances and make an effort to know people. But in high school, it's a rare person indeed who grasps this concept; rarer still is the young man or woman who embraces it as a way of life. In high school, popularity is rooted in physical appearance. And I was fortunate.

In some ways this caused a conflict for me. Growing up in a Chinese-American family, I was taught humility as well as pride. My parents expected their children to excel, to work hard, and be the best they could possibly be, especially in the classroom. Recognition from outsiders, though, was viewed with skepticism, especially when it stemmed largely from something so frivolous as popularity and looks. Our family was quiet, reserved, and wary of attention. But I liked the attention. When I became the first female, and the first Asian-American, to be elected student body vice-president, I was thrilled.

Interestingly, there was only one other Asian person in my entire high school, but I never sensed any different treatment. Maybe that's because even though I looked Chinese, and at home we embraced many Chinese traditions and mores, I sounded very American. I looked like an American kid. I wanted the things other American kids wanted. In the fall of my senior year, for example, I was one of four nominees for homecoming queen. The other girls were all close friends of mine, and I was happy to be sharing the honor and the excitement with them. But like any other American teenager I would be lying if I said I didn't want to win. Homecoming was held at the Bakersfield Junior College football stadium, which sat nineteen thousand people. As tradition dictated, the coronation was conducted at halftime of our game against Bakersfield High School. When my name was announced as the winner, and I was crowned homecoming queen, well . . . all I can say is that every person should experience such a wonderful feeling.

A couple of months later I attended the Foothill High School Christmas Formal, escorted by an exchange student from Thailand. It was so much fun getting all dressed up, picking out a gown with my mom, getting pinned with a corsage. I was on the decoration committee, too, so I put a lot of work into the event. Mainly, though, it was just fun. The highlight of the evening was the announcement of the Christmas Formal Queen. Having already been homecoming queen, I certainly didn't expect to get another crown on this night. So as I was standing in the back of the room, and my name was called, I was almost too stunned to move. People were pushing me, telling me to go up on stage, applauding and patting me on the back. I remember grabbing my date and saying, "You're going up there with me." We walked to the stage together, and if my initial reaction was one of embarrassment, it quickly dissolved into pride as the music played and we danced a solo dance for the entire ballroom.

The wonderful things I was fortunate enough to experience as a teenager helped give me a unique perspective. I've been a homecoming queen and an adult woman with a disability so severe that people sometimes averted their glance. The world works in strange ways.

Beauty may be only skin deep, but a lot of people have trouble getting past the skin. When you're young, and especially when you're female, you're trained to believe that physical appearance goes a long way toward determining your happiness and success. It's certainly not what I believe today, but as a young woman it was all I knew. My beliefs about beauty then were guided (even subconsciously directed) by TV, magazines, the movies, and my friends. Today, while I still try to do the best with what I've been given (good or bad), I have learned that real beauty bubbles up from the inside out. Unless you give others a chance to see your internal beauty, they will judge you based on what they see externally. In my struggle with the deformities of crippling arthritis and how it repulsed people around me, I withdrew into myself. I didn't like myself because others didn't like the way I looked. It took me many years to figure out that I could actually change the deep sadness I experienced from being so deformed and "ugly." I decided to focus on the things I could control, building up and pushing out my inner reservoir of personality, dynamism, humor, communication skills, kindness, grace, and a magnetism stronger than physical appearance—my own sense of optimism and hope.

There is no small irony in the timing of the onset of my illness. It started during my last two years in high school, at a time when I felt pretty good about myself. I had no idea what was happening, and really had no reason to believe anything sinister was at work deep in my body. I was getting sick a lot. I'd catch a cold or a nasty case of the flu, and eventually it would develop into something more serious, like mononucleosis. What was happening, I later discovered, was that my whole immune system was going haywire. I felt tired, feverish, I ached all over. First my toes would be sore, then my knees and elbows. Sometimes my ears would feel hot. I wouldn't describe any of it as "pain." It was more of a soreness and a general feeling of lethargy. When you're a kid, though, you dismiss these things pretty quickly. You get sick, you bounce back, you get on with your life.

It wasn't until my freshman year in college, at the University of California at Santa Barbara, that I became aware of the seriousness of my condition. The first alarm was a persistent pain in my sternum, an ache that seemed disconnected from any previous ailment. I remember sitting at my desk in my dorm room one night, doing homework, and reaching for a stack of papers. The ache was suddenly replaced by a sharp pain, as if someone had punched me in my chest, near my heart. My breath hitched for a moment and I thought, *Wow! What was that?* The pain subsided, though, and I passed it off as a side effect of too much exercise. I'd been swimming a lot, playing golf, tennis, and generally just enjoying the seaside ambience that makes UCSB one of the greatest places in the world to attend college. I shuffled my papers and went back to work. A few minutes later, when I leaned over again, the pain came back, stronger and sharper this time. I let out a little whimper and felt a surge of panic.

Oh, my God! Am I having a heart attack or something?

But once again the pain receded. I decided to take a nice warm shower and go to bed. In the morning, I thought, everything would be fine. I'd take the day off from working out, give my muscles a chance to recover, and soon I'd be as good as new.

It didn't work out that way. When I woke, the pain had returned. This time it was steady and hard, as if someone were squeezing my heart. I should have gone straight to the campus hospital, but I didn't. After all, I was a college freshman, which means I existed somewhere in that nebulous state between childhood and adulthood. Away from home for the very first time, sharing a room with someone I barely knew, trying to find my way in the world, I was adamant about solving my own problems. The last thing I wanted to do was cry out for help, and I sure wasn't going to pick up the phone and call my parents. No, instead, I sat on my bed for a little while, got my breathing under control, and took another shower. Then I dressed and went off to class, biting my lip to fight the pain the entire time.

For a long time I didn't tell anyone what I was going through, primarily because I just couldn't imagine there was anything seriously wrong with me. I was young, healthy, active, and I was having a great time in college. Even though I was only a freshman, I was voted president of the largest women's dormitory on campus. I joined a forensics club to sharpen my oratory skills. I was doing well in all of my classes. I was making lots of new friends. All these accomplishments served to dull the impact of the pain I was feeling. My strategy, if you can call it that, was simply this: keep moving, keep moving, keep moving. The pain would ebb and flow, and I found that by distracting myself with activities I could lessen the impact of the occasional flare (although, at the time, I didn't even know what a flare was).

Eventually, I told my parents what was happening, although only because I was going home for a weekend and I knew there was no way I was going to be able to keep it from them. They'd see me wincing, holding my chest, and the secret would be out. Better to tell them before I arrived, I reasoned. Predictably, their response was to call Uncle Eugene, an internal medicine doctor. My mother never wanted to see the doctor herself, but she wasn't going to let her daughter get away with a similarly cavalier attitude. So, that weekend, I drove to Uncle Eugene's office in Fresno. He gave me a complete physical, poked me and prodded me, and came to the following conclusion: "You've been playing too much tennis. You probably strained a muscle."

Well, that was a relief. A strained muscle would heal. Since it was my uncle offering the diagnosis, a man who had known me since I was a baby, and who knew my entire family history, I was certain that I had nothing to worry about.

"We're going to give you a little shot of cortisone in your chest," he said. "It'll help you feel better."

"Whatever you say, Uncle Eugene."

If you've ever received an injection of cortisone, you know there is no such thing as "a little shot." In my memory the needle is about eighteen inches long (in reality it was probably about six inches) and filled with battery acid. I nearly passed out from the injection.

"Close your eyes, Amye," Uncle Eugene had said. "This won't hurt."

He was trying to assuage my fears. But as the needle went in, my chest filled with fire. Uncle Eugene literally had to pin me down to complete the process. Fortunately, he was quick—it was over in a matter of seconds.

"Okay," he said. "I know that was rough. Just close your eyes and rest. Go to sleep if you'd like."

I didn't sleep, but I did let my mind drift. That was the very first time I used digression to cope with something unpleasant. I stared up at the ceiling, a textured surface with thousands of airholes for sound absorption, and tried to count the little dots, just to see if it would take my mind off the pain. It worked, too, at least a little bit. This type of disassociation has served me well over the years in dealing with pain. The mind is an amazing thing, and the more you can harness its recuperative powers, the better equipped you'll be to deal with arthritis or any other chronic illness. Digression can be something as simple as watching (I mean really *focusing on*) a TV program, a movie, even the words to a song. By directing your attention to something interesting, thought provoking, or pleasant, you give your body and emotions a reprieve from the pain of the moment.

The cortisone worked with predictable alacrity and efficiency . . . at first. After about three days, however, the pain came back. It came back with such thunderous force that I called Uncle Eugene and went straight to his office. This time he wasn't nearly as calm and reassuring.

"Something's wrong," he said. "This shouldn't be happening."

One of the problems with rheumatoid arthritis is that, in its early stages, it can be a highly difficult disease to diagnose. The symptoms mimic any number of other injuries and illnesses, and so it becomes a process of elimination. There is no single test you can take that will instantly light up a strip of litmus paper with the words *You've got it—rheumatoid arthritis!* It's really a combination of several clinical evaluations by an experienced doctor. There are blood tests now that will confirm or deny the Rh factor and give you an idea of whether you have a predisposition to rheumatoid antibodies in your system, but that's about the extent of it. And, naturally, arthritis is just about the last thing you'd look for in an otherwise healthy, active eighteen-year-old woman—even if the doctor is married to a woman who suffers from the disease. That's right. Uncle Eugene was married to Martha, a beautiful Italian woman with rheumatoid arthritis! He witnessed the effects of this disease every day when he went home from the office, and yet it didn't occur to him that I might have the same thing. That's how mysterious and misunderstood a disease arthritis can be.

In time, though, a conclusion was reached. Uncle Eugene called me one day, and we met at his office.

"Amye," he said calmly, his voice not betraying the gravity of the situation. "We know what's causing your pain."

I leaned forward, more curious than concerned. "That's good. Tell me what it is."

"You have something known as rheumatoid arthritis."

I was perplexed. My mind processed only half of the diagnosis: the word *arthritis*.

"Uncle Eugene, what are you talking about? Isn't arthritis for old people?"

He shook his head. "Not necessarily. We're talking about a different kind of arthritis. The good news is, we can treat it. We'll give you a lot of medication, and that will minimize the symptoms. You'll be all right."

We hugged, and I left the office. Then I drove back home, still largely oblivious to the severity of the diagnosis I'd just been handed. Arthritis, to me, was canes and crutches and wheelchairs. It was little old people bent over and shuffling along. It had nothing to do with me. I was laboring under a misconception that hasn't changed even today. As I was about to discover, arthritis is not just for old people.

3

Image Is Everything

I remember as a little girl seeing television advertisements in which an older person would be depicted as moving a little slowly, maybe rubbing an elbow or shoulder. The voice-over would say something like "Take aspirin . . . for the minor aches and pains of arthritis." My reaction then was one of naive sympathy and optimism: *This is a condition of old age, but at least you can do something about it. Isn't that nice?*

When I was hit with a diagnosis of arthritis, my whole outlook changed. I was upset on several levels. One, the image of arthritis presented in that commercial was not me, and yet I had been given a sentence of arthritis. Two, the advertisement recommended taking aspirin for arthritis, and although one of the first therapies prescribed for my arthritis was aspirin, it certainly was not in the dosages casually mentioned in this commercial. I was popping twenty-six aspirin a day! And number three, the part about "minor aches and pains." The assumption seemed to be that arthritis pain was, by definition, "minor," when in fact what I was experiencing was quite severe. There were times when I could barely get out of a chair, when I had trouble walking across a room. *Minor?* I don't think so.

The contradiction between what I saw on television and what I was experiencing in my own life, in my own body, created a good deal of emotional turmoil. I began to question my own strength. I wondered if I was imagining the pain in my knees and hands. Something was very wrong, because the way arthritis was affecting me was nothing like the image presented on television. *I'm not old. I'm young! And yet, in a lot of ways, I look just like that white-haired woman shuffling slowly down the sidewalk.* As I continued to investigate, I discovered that the misconceptions related to arthritis were not only profound but also pervasive. After all, everybody knows somebody who has arthritis: an aunt or an uncle or a grandmother or a grandfather. So the prevailing attitude is *It's just part of old age—what's the big deal?*

This attitude, which represents a trivializing of the effects of the illness, often has a dramatic impact on the person who suffers from arthritis, especially if that person is young. You try to hide the symptoms. You go out of your way not to talk about it, because every time someone asks you why you're moving a little slowly, why you're grimacing, and you say, "Oh, I've got arthritis," the response is something like "Yeah, I know what you mean. I've got a sore elbow and the doctor tells me I should stop playing tennis for a few weeks." Equating tennis elbow to rheumatoid arthritis, or advanced osteoarthritis, or lupus is ludicrous, and yet it happens all the time. There's nothing malicious about it, of course; it's just a matter of ignorance. But when it persists, it can really beat you down.

Arthritis truly is a hidden disability. Even though I had a firm diagnosis of rheumatoid arthritis with accompanying pain, fatigue, and stilted movements, I found myself having to prove to people around me that I was indeed suffering. Initially, arthritis has no badge of identification to the outside world, no crutches or leg cast that automatically tells the world, "Be careful around me; I hurt." Not until I was forced to use crutches and later landed in a wheel-chair did people begin to see that I was truly suffering. And then it seemed the whole world became more sensitive to my needs: open-ing heavy doors, helping me find chairs, offering to carry heavy groceries. Funny thing is, I hadn't changed. The arthritis pain was there all along.

The relative invisibility of the disease in its earliest stages can be equally hard on your self-esteem and psyche. You may walk kind of funny, you hurt, your energy level is low, but there really isn't an ob-vious sign announcing to the world that you have a disease. Sadly, but perhaps understandably, people judge you on the basis of what they see. They can tell something is bothering you, but they don't know what. People would often say to me, "What's wrong, Amye?" When I would respond, "I have arthritis," people would dismiss it completely. It was frustrating. You have to explain to people why you have a limp, or why you can't turn your head to the side, or why you can't play tennis anymore. You have to explain that persistent pain is making you irritable, moody. You have to do this because you are not what society expects of a sick person. They want to see the cast or the scars or the hospital visit to validate how they should react to you. In the beginning, though, I had none of the outward symptoms of an ill woman. That's the way it is for most people with arthritis.

Very soon after my diagnosis, I stopped telling people what was affecting me. If they saw me limping and inquired as to the reason, I'd tell them I'd been involved in a skiing accident, or something like that. Anything was better than hearing people compare my condi-tion to their mild tendinitis, or, worse, hearing them say, incredu-lously, usually with a dismissive wave of the hand, "Oh, come on, you're way too young to have arthritis." It seemed as though if you were under fifty years of age, you were immune to the ravages of this disease. Certainly when you're eighteen or nineteen, as I was, it's inconceivable to most people that you could be stricken by an illness that nearly everyone associates with the elderly. The feedback you're getting is (a) you're a liar or (b) you're a freak. Either way, it's an unpleasant response. Pretty soon, after you've met enough resistance, you get wise. You learn how to tell little white lies. That's what I did. I became a very good storyteller. A consequence of lying to others, however, is that you're also lying to yourself. You don't face the situation. You don't go to the doctor as often as you should. You don't seek treatment. You tell yourself you're all right, when in reality you're on a downward spiral.

At first it seems like the easy way out, but in reality, you're digging yourself in deeper. Arthritis affects every aspect of your life, including how you protect yourself from and project yourself to others. The longer you avoid facing up to the reality of what arthritis is or what it can do to you, the more you allow it to beat you down. I allowed arthritis to consume my every thought, belief, and action. The end result was that I hid. I hid my emotions and fears. I didn't like what I saw in the mirror—the reflection of how I moved or functioned. I especially didn't like the pity innocently bestowed on me by others.

What I know today is that the best strategy for dealing with arthritis is to study the disease and stand up to it. That's called taking charge, getting control, and managing your health and well-being. It took me years to figure this out by reading voraciously about arthritis and arthritis management, the psychology of chronic disease, changing attitudes and behaviors, meditation and focusing, humor, goal setting, and communicating with others. Today, the Arthritis Foundation in the United States has excellent education and management programs that incorporate these important concepts to help people and families affected by arthritis learn to regain control of their lives.

I've learned that when it comes to image, communication is the key element for a person with arthritis. It has to start and end with you. Today, when a stranger asks "What's wrong with you?" my response doesn't just end with "I have arthritis." Instead, I gear it toward function by saying, "I have something called rheumatoid arthritis, and the pain in my knees and hands makes it painful to walk and open doors, so thanks for holding the door open for me!" I try to end my comments with a gracious smile and gratitude for having the stranger do something that might seem trivial to him or her but is a great help to me. This kind of communication gives just enough information to satisfy a curious stranger, and keeps you in control by connecting the image of arthritis to specific functional difficulties you may have.

People with arthritis are stigmatized. I know that might sound strange if you've never experienced the quizzical looks and skeptical responses, but it's true. When you think of being stigmatized, you probably think of AIDS, or maybe cancer twenty years ago. Arthritis has a stigma attached to it that is not so much about death as it is about age, about being old. *Old* is a word we don't like in our society, for it implies not only that death is near but also that a sense of purpose and value has been lost. In our society, being old is not cool. Being old is not being vibrant. Being old means being dependent. To a young person diagnosed with arthritis, the flood of images is overwhelming. Worse than being sick is the notion that you are not what you thought you were. Funny, isn't it? When you're a gangly adolescent of thirteen or fourteen, a jumble of pubescent angst and energy, you can't wait to be older. As childhood recedes and you head into your twenties or thirties, you'd just as soon have the clock slow down a bit. To be suddenly trapped inside a body that feels ninety-five years old . . . well, that's a terrifying proposition; worse is the fear that others will *see* you as a ninety-five-year-old woman.

When all these feelings converged on me at once, the effect was, to say the least, traumatic. It might as well have been cancer. In fact, in some ways, it was worse, because I suffered alone. There were no support groups for teenagers with rheumatoid arthritis, no one with whom I could share my fears and insecurities. My response was to go into denial, to pretend I wasn't really sick.

Today, I counsel a lot of young people about this attitude, which means, unfortunately, that things haven't changed all that much in terms of perception. But the resources available now are much more pervasive. Through patient organizations like the Arthritis Foundation and credible websites, support groups, news groups, and chat sessions, young adults can easily get access to good-quality information, meet others in similar situations, and take a big first step toward avoiding the loneliness and isolation so often associated with young adults and arthritis.

Arthritis is still generally viewed as a disease of the aged. Indeed, there are some types of arthritis that afflict the elderly in far greater numbers than any other group, but it's important to understand that the disease has many different faces. When most people use the word *"arthritis,"* they are talking about osteoarthritis or degenerative joint disease, which is clearly associated with the aging process. Chances are, if you are graced with a long life, you will eventually feel the effects of osteoarthritis. What happens is this: Through general wear and tear, the cartilage in a joint (and this can be any joint—elbow, knee, spine, shoulder, even fingers and toes) begins to deteriorate. When the cartilage is damaged in any way, when there is even the slightest disruption in the joint, the body compensates and you begin to move it differently, and thus begins the degenerative process, one that feeds on itself. Instead of having nice, smooth, well-rounded joint cartilage, you have something that looks like a bald or pitted tire. The joint wears unevenly, pieces of bone and cartilage are sheared off, and before long the integrity of the joint is compromised.

The deterioration of the joint can be fast or slow, but the end result is that you stop moving that joint because of pain. In some
cases the entire process is accelerated as a result of a traumatic injury—an automobile accident, for instance, or, more commonly,
an athletic injury. Athletes are more prone to osteoarthritis because of overuse. If you're a quarterback, it isn't just getting
creamed by a linebacker and drilled into the turf that makes you a
likely candidate for arthritis; it's the fact that every day you are putting tremendous stress on all your joints. Think of it like this: Ge-
netically, maybe you're supposed to move a specific joint one
million times over the course of your lifetime. The average person
is well into his sixties or seventies before he reaches that number;
however, the athlete hits one million by the time he's thirty-five
years old, which naturally quickens the demise of his joint.

Although it is the most common form, osteoarthritis is merely
one type of arthritis. The diseases of the musculoskeletal system, in
fact, constitute a fairly large and extended family. Rheumatoid
arthritis (with which I am personally familiar) is a systemic disease,
affecting the entire body, and as such is one of the most crippling
forms of arthritis. Rheumatoid arthritis affects organs as well as
joints, although it is typically experienced as a maddeningly painful
and debilitating disease that robs the individual of the ability to use
her joints in a normal manner. In rheumatoid arthritis it is the joint
fluid and lining, as well as the cartilage, that is affected. We don't
know why yet. We know only that something in the body's immune
system has gone completely haywire, resulting in a cannibalistic
process: the body turns on itself, with antibodies attacking healthy
cells and destroying a perfectly vital joint. The synovial fluid that
lines the joints, that protects the ends of the joints, and that should
be clear and smooth, like corn syrup, becomes murky, like sludge.
It's like a car: when the oil gets mucky, the engine can be seriously
damaged. Synovial fluid affected by rheumatoid arthritis literally
eats away at whatever it touches—first cartilage, then bone, finally

muscle. The entire joint space decreases in size, and the person experiences excruciating pain. Unfortunately, with rheumatoid arthritis, there's no way to change the oil. Once the synovial fluid is seriously damaged, there's not much that can be done. A number of drugs have been used in an attempt to slow or reverse the process, but none has been completely effective yet. (Some newer drugs are now available in the United States and Europe that show promise.) And, unfortunately, by the time most patients are diagnosed, their joints may have already been significantly compromised.

Rheumatoid arthritis is even less predictable than osteoarthritis. It can move quickly or slowly. It can affect one joint or twenty. It can be mildly debilitating or virtually crippling. When you are first diagnosed, there is no way to know where the road will lead. As with any type of arthritis, though, early intervention by an arthritis specialist, a rheumatologist, is essential to maintaining some semblance of a healthy, active life. Generally speaking, rheumatoid arthritis moves like a large predator, feeding on the biggest joints (hips, shoulders, knees) before moving on to the joints in the hands and feet. It affects women in far greater numbers than men (women are two to three times more likely to develop rheumatoid arthritis). Medical science has yet to come up with an explanation for this disparity, although there seems to be some sort of a hormonal connection. Ironically, one piece of advice given to many women who suffer from rheumatoid arthritis is "Get pregnant!" I had one doctor offer that piece of advice to me. He called me into his office and, with a big smile, said, "Amye, I know what you can do to get rid of your rheumatoid arthritis."

Excited almost beyond words, I fairly gushed, "What? Tell me!"

"Have a baby!"

"Excuse me?"

Was this guy kidding? I was in so much pain I could barely manage a sexual relationship. How was I going to take care of a baby? And what exactly was the science behind this theory, anyway?

"When women get pregnant," he explained, "their rheumatoid arthritis usually goes into remission. More than that, even. The symptoms disappear completely . . . "

He paused. *Bombshell coming.*

". . . for a while."

"Uh-huh. But it comes back, right?"

"Well, yes. It may eventually."

Oh, great, I thought. *So what do I do with the baby? You know—the result of this pregnancy? Who would take care of the little guy?* This doctor hadn't given much thought to that part of the equation. Still, for some women it is an option. Something about pregnancy is wonderful for battling rheumatoid arthritis. If you have the proper support system, maybe it's worth it. The downside, of course, is that the symptoms may return.

It's not an easy choice.

There are numerous other diseases you might not typically associate with arthritis but that are, in fact, closely related. Fibromyalgia, for example. A lot of people with fibromyalgia don't think of it as arthritis because it doesn't directly affect the joints, but it is considered in the arthritis family. It's characterized by pain in the muscles and fibrous connective tissue (tendons and ligaments). More so than with osteoarthritis or rheumatoid arthritis, which are typified by persistent, throbbing pain over a fairly widespread area, fibromyalgia is characterized by tender points, specific areas of the body that are intensely sensitive to the touch. As a result, fibromyalgia results in extreme fatigue and lack of good-quality deep sleep.

Another not uncommon type of musculoskeletal disease is lupus, which can affect the joints, heart, lungs, kidneys, central nervous system, and the skin. More than 80 percent of all persons diagnosed with lupus are women, and a large percentage of these are African-American. Symptoms of lupus include fatigue, fever, skin rash, muscle aches, nausea, swollen glands, sensitivity to cold, weight loss, sensitivity to the sun, and pain and stiffness in the joints.

Like lupus, scleroderma (which is Greek for "hard skin") affects internal organs and the skin. Another example of the body's autoimmune system backfiring, scleroderma can be a terrifically painful and disfiguring disease in which the skin becomes thick and hard, resulting in an almost reptilian appearance. But the damage is far worse than what is visible to the naked eye, for scleroderma progresses from the outside in, eventually attacking the esophagus, kidneys, heart, lungs, and intestinal tract. It's a brutal disease that, like most musculoskeletal ailments, affects more women than men.

Another member of this family of diseases is juvenile rheumatoid arthritis (JRA). In many ways, JRA is like rheumatoid arthritis, except that it affects children under the age of eighteen, as young as one to two months of age, and is more commonly associated with dangerously high fevers. We don't think of young people, even young adults, as suffering from arthritis, and we certainly don't think of children as being affected; the truth, however, is that more than three hundred thousand children in the United States alone have JRA. That's a phenomenal number—greater in fact, than the number of children diagnosed with cystic fibrosis. And yet we devote more research dollars to cystic fibrosis (and have a far greater understanding of the disease) than we do to JRA. Is that because cystic fibrosis is a known killer, a disease that almost always takes the lives of its victims at some point? Perhaps. I'm certainly not going to suggest that we shouldn't be pumping tons of money into finding a cure for cystic fibrosis; I'm simply saying that children with juvenile rheumatoid arthritis suffer terribly, and I've counseled a lot of young people who have shared with me that their suffering is so great that they longed for death, and in fact were considering suicide. Children and young adults with arthritis, and anyone else afflicted with any of the more than one hundred different types of arthritis, deserve better; they deserve to have a better quality of life; they deserve *hope*.

There are many reasons why we have yet to find a cure for arthritis. In part, the problem lies in the complexity of the disease, the fact that it has so many faces and forms. It is a mysterious disease whose path is rarely straight and narrow; rather, it twists and turns, rises and falls. A diagnosis is barely the beginning, for even with a diagnosis there is no way to know which course the disease will take, how it will manifest itself, or how severe a particular case will be. So there is the enigmatic nature of the disease to overcome.

As I've said, though, a far more significant obstacle is the perception that arthritis is merely an inconvenience, a perfectly normal and acceptable part of the aging process that can be dealt with effectively through the use of aspirin and other over-the-counter medications. In other words, it's just not a sexy disease, and therefore not sufficiently compelling to attract vast piles of research dollars. It's perceived as not being as intriguing as AIDS or cancer or any number of other diseases more likely to merit significant government funding or contributions from the public. Arthritis is too often the victim of the "squeaky wheel" syndrome: when there is significant advocacy and a large enough population of young people at risk (as is the case with AIDS), the federal government begins to listen and, more important, applies resources to groups interested in eradicating the problem. It's a fact of life: politicians listen when the power of the vote becomes apparent. What is remarkable is that the arthritis community has the potential to flex more muscle than any other afflicted group. We are talking about 43 million people in the United States alone! That is a vast and powerful constituency, and I believe it is only a matter of time before we are given the support and respect we deserve.

Again, please don't misunderstand me. I'm not for a moment suggesting we should cut funding for AIDS or cancer research. I'm simply saying more money and effort should be devoted to arthritis research. I've always believed (and there is a sizable chunk of the scientific community that agrees) that when we find a cure for AIDS, we will go a long way toward finding a cure for other diseases like rheumatoid arthritis, lupus, and scleroderma, because they're all diseases that affect the immune system. There has to be a link.

The best weapons currently at our disposal can be effective, but vary from person to person. Anti-inflammatory drugs can help with the pain; newer drugs, such as the COX-2 inhibitors, have been shown to help reduce inflammation in osteoarthritis and rheumatoid arthritis; and biologic response modifiers can change the course of rheumatoid arthritis.

But there is no cure . . . yet.

If society's attitude toward arthritis hasn't changed much, at least the medical field's approach to attacking the disease has become more aggressive and enlightened. When I was first diagnosed, the doctors would start by prescribing aspirin and gradually build up to stronger and more toxic drugs. Today it's completely reversed. The philosophy is "Let's not start with the small stuff just because we're afraid of toxicity; let's go right to the big guns to get the disease under control as soon as possible." The reason for this change is simple: We don't know enough about arthritis, and we don't have a cure yet; what we do know is that if we don't treat it early and aggressively, then we're not just looking at pain, we're looking at long-term disability. Then the costs for the person affected, her family, and society are enormous.

In regard to medications, the doctors always used to say, "We're concerned with Amye's stomach, we're concerned with Amye's hair falling out . . . " Yes, arthritis medications can be toxic, but the trade-off is improved quality of life. I was in constant flare with symptoms that kept getting worse. Arthritis, especially rheumatoid arthritis, is like a wildfire, and if the firefighters don't contain the blaze quickly, it's going to spread. In the early days of my arthritis, precious little was known about controlling arthritis. The doctors just wanted to make sure I didn't develop ulcers from taking too much medication. In fairness, I have to say that some of the treatments were dangerous, and some trepidation on the part of my physicians was warranted. In my heart, though, I believe that it's better to be aggressive than passive in treating almost any form of arthritis, and I'm not alone. Today, the medical community realizes that arthritis is the number-one cause of workplace disability for a reason. It has this dubious distinction because it prevents people from moving, from working, from leading productive lives. Now, if we can only get the politicians who fund arthritis research to see the misconceptions caused by the image of arthritis!

In the progression of the disease, the pain that comes with erosion of joint padding, and a subsequent lessening of joint space, can be intense. I equate it to a door jamb. In order for the hinge to work properly, the door has to be set slightly apart from the frame. When the door expands or moves out of line and gets too close to the frame, what happens? The door won't work properly. It won't close tightly or it won't open all the way. There is constant rubbing, grinding, and irritation. Now, imagine that there are thousands of hypersensitive little nerve fibers all along the edge of the door, right at the contact point, and you get the idea. The joint, where the ends of two bones come together, is moving all the time, and with each movement, the irritation and erosion increase. Besides muscles, tendons, and ligaments, the joint is surrounded by nerves, like the pulp of a tooth. You know what happens with a cavity when the pulp is exposed? Well, when the cartilage in a joint wears away, and bone meets bone, with nerve endings brushing up against one another, the sharp pain is excruciating. More than that, actually. In severe cases of osteoarthritis and rheumatoid arthritis, the pain can be downright unbearable.

The human body really is a wondrous mechanism, intricately and uniquely designed for movement. We are not meant to be sedentary. When we stop moving, pieces of the machine begin to falter. Muscles atrophy, joints stiffen, and organs work less effectively. It's a sad paradox faced by the person with arthritis: the body has to move in order to work efficiently and gain nutrients, but pain makes that movement difficult, if not impossible; the mind fairly screams at the body, "*Stop!*" Pain dictates everything about arthritis, and you have to somehow learn to deal with it. If you move too much, you do damage; if you move too little, you wither away. It's a fine line that must be walked . . . if you want to keep on walking.

The end result with degenerative destructive arthritis, whether it's rheumatoid or osteoarthritis, is a joint so ravaged that it must be replaced. This is what happened to me, only a lot faster than it typically happens to most people with arthritis. The ideal candidate for joint replacement surgery is someone in her middle to late sixties. By that time you've slowed down a lot, and you're putting less stress on your joints. There are exceptions, of course, but most people of that age are not running marathons, jumping out of airplanes, or climbing Himalayan peaks. They are still young enough to lead healthy, active lives, but not so young that they're going to put undue stress on their joints. And, to add a rather blunt footnote, they're not so young that they're going to outlive the joint replacement. You have to understand, the whole idea of a joint replacement is to make sure the prosthesis lasts longer than the body in which it is housed. When I started asking my doctors, "What will it take to get me out of a wheelchair?" their response was, "You need joint replacements. Unfortunately, you're too young."

I was incredulous. "Too young for what?! When will I be old enough?"

"Uhhh . . . when you're in your fifties or sixties."

This made no sense to me. "I have to wait thirty years to be a candidate for surgery that will allow me to walk? Do you know what I'll look like by then? Do you know what my life will be like—if I'm even alive?"

But they didn't get it. It was all about making sure the joint replacement would be viable and last long enough to be considered a "success." Joint replacements typically have a life span of about fifteen years, depending on the joint. From the orthopedic surgeon's point of view, a joint replacement candidate in her late twenties, as I was, is about as bad an investment as you can make. Eventually all my replacements will fail, and I'll have to go through the whole process all over again. That's the price I have to pay, and I am willing to pay it. I was willing to bet on technology giving me a better life, rather than waiting thirty years to be a candidate for surgery that might no longer even be relevant or viable for me. Guaranteeing a positive result was not my top priority; I just wanted a fighting chance. Finding a doctor, or a team of doctors, who was equally motivated and enthusiastic was no small task.

I wish I had known then what I know today about how to find and communicate with a physician. I wasn't sure of myself then. And although I knew I needed help from a medical professional, I didn't know what kind of professional relationship I needed in order to bring clarity to medically or surgically managing my arthritis. Understanding the kind of person you are and the type of information you need to make the most appropriate decisions about your health are the first steps to learning how to communicate with your physician. It starts with you, not your physician. Are you the kind of person who wants to know the details of tests, or how medications and treatment impact your disease process? Or are you the kind of person who prefers to leave all the details to your physician and just be told what to do? Knowing how deeply you want to be involved in medical discussions and decisions is integral to finding the best physician for you.

Once you understand how the image of arthritis affects the way people react to you, you're a step farther down the road. Let your words be the lasting impression of anyone who meets you, not the way you walk. Anticipate their comments and be prepared to counter them and even educate them.

In advocating for proper treatment with your doctor, tie how you feel to specific functions. When your physician asks how you are at the start of your visit, remember that this is not a social question. This is an entrée for you to state your concerns. For example, instead of stating "I hurt all the time," consider the specifics. Try to find the appropriate words to describe how you feel, when the pain intensifies, what activities you do or can't do because of your pain, what therapies you've tried to reduce it, and its frequency. Become a partner with your doctor so that together you can find the best treatment for you.

In my research I discovered an interesting thing about that television commercial, the one in which aspirin was recommended for the "minor aches and pains of arthritis." The reason it was worded in such an awkward, misleading way is that there were (and are) communication regulations restricting false or overly optimistic advertising. It was a way to ensure that the manufacturers didn't claim that their product (in this case aspirin) had any great curative effect on more severe types of arthritis. Logical, and perhaps rooted in the best of intentions, these restrictions nonetheless perpetuated a myth about arthritis: that it is nothing more than a minor ailment, and a natural component of the aging process that can be cured with simple aspirin. My dad used to watch this commercial and just shake his head.

"Hah!" he'd say. *"Minor aches and pains . . .* If they could only see my daughter."

4

Denial: Not Just a River in Egypt

One of the more interesting and disorienting things about the onset of sudden, chronic illness is that you are instantly thrust into a strange, new world. It's a world full of doctors and nurses and pills, all of which are supposed to be helping. Sometimes, though, their plan doesn't work, and you continue to spiral downward. Instead of feeling better, you're feeling worse. I had never been really sick prior to being diagnosed with arthritis. Sick, to me, meant catching a cold, spending a day or two in bed with the flu, maybe having chicken pox or measles. Being sick meant a few days of discomfort, a prescription for an antibiotic, and then feeling good as new. None of these experiences had in any way prepared me for the overwhelming effect that rheumatoid arthritis would have on every facet of my life. I was eighteen years old and had just been told that I was going to be sick for the rest of my days. That was the underlying message, anyway. What I heard was something more like this: *"You have arthritis and we'll treat it with medication and you'll be fine."*

Placed on a therapy whose foundation was an astounding twenty-six aspirin a day, I quickly discovered that managing my arthritis was going to be a bit more complicated than I had envisioned. Whether I was home or at school, out socializing with friends or at my desk doing my homework, I always had to be aware of the time so that I could take my medication on schedule. Because aspirin is highly acidic and can cause ulcers, I had to drink of a lot of liquid, usually milk, which buffered the corrosive qualities of the aspirin. As a consequence, I spent considerable time running back and forth to the bathroom. Maintaining this schedule was particularly difficult at night, when I had to set an alarm so that I'd wake up every four hours. Each night before I went to bed I'd put a bottle of milk in a bowl of ice and place it on my nightstand, not only to save time, but to save energy as well. There were nights, even in the beginning, when I was so tired that I didn't have the strength to get out of bed. If you have arthritis, you know exactly what I'm talking about. But if you don't, this probably sounds ridiculous. I understand that. I absolutely do. How could anyone who hasn't experienced this disease possibly know how difficult it was for me to sit up in bed, swing my legs out over the side of the bed, put my feet on the floor, and walk to the bathroom in the middle of the night, when my joints were virtually locked in place? It sounds absurd, especially coming from a vibrant, athletic teenager. That's one of the things that makes arthritis such an exhausting and frustrating disease: no one understands what you're going through; quite often, they think you're faking, looking for sympathy.

Complicating matters, and deepening my confusion, was the fact that my primary medication was nothing more than aspirin. How sick could I be? After all, I'd been taking aspirin since I was a kid. Hadn't everyone? Granted, very few people know what it's like to gobble twenty-six tablets a day, but still, if I'd been handed a death sentence, or a sentence of progressive deterioration, ending in invalidism, wouldn't they be doing . . . I don't know . . . *more?*

Well, no. This was nearly twenty-five years ago, practically a lifetime in medical science, and while it may have been the Stone Age when compared to twenty-first-century care, it also reflected the conventional wisdom of the time. Aspirin therapy was the first step in a long course of treatment, the toxicity and aggressiveness of which would be increased only when previous steps had failed. Try explaining any of that to your college roommate when you're eighteen years old. There was nothing malicious about my first college roomie, nothing hostile or even slightly prejudicial. She was just oblivious. She saw me as a healthy young woman. When I tried to explain to her what I was going through, she seemed confused.

"Then why are they only giving you aspirin?"

I really had no plausible answer. After all, her question was my question, and it was a question I faced from numerous other students during my college career. After a while I just shut down. I began to get quiet, at least on the subject of arthritis. It wasn't a conscious effort—it just sort of happened, because I got tired of fighting. Through my work today as a peer counselor and public speaker, I've come into contact with people with arthritis who have experienced exactly this same response. What happens is, when people ask you a question, instead of answering in one hundred words, you answer in twenty words, then in ten. You give them the least amount of information required to make them go away. In time, you become an island. It's just you and arthritis—a messy, miserable, dysfunctional little couple.

Today I look back at those times and see how I was shutting down. I couldn't face the disease myself, so how was I going to project it to others? What would have been more helpful was to confide in the friends and instructors closest to me. Asking for their help when I needed it, and having their support, would have given me greater emotional relief. So much of what I know now could have changed the decisions I made about the course of my disease then.

As much as possible, I tried to compartmentalize my rheumatoid arthritis. It wasn't hard to figure out that on any college campus, including UCSB, it's possible to reinvent yourself—over and over. You can make new friends, develop new interests. You can be anything you want to be. As long as I didn't discuss it, as long as I didn't complain too loudly or end up having such a terrible flare that I needed hospitalization, I didn't have to be a young person with arthritis. I could just live with it. It was my business, and nobody else's.

Or so I thought.

This philosophy served me well for a while. I was elected president of the largest women's dorm in my freshman year—in part, I think, because I was the only candidate who created a logo for her campaign posters. (I chose a ladybug, because according to Chinese tradition, ladybugs are a sign of good luck.) In retrospect, I know that I ran for this position not only because I wanted the job, but also because it allowed me to focus on something other than my arthritis.

As much as it is an academic and educational experience, college is a social experience. It represents an opportunity to act like an adult, but in a playful setting. You're making your own decisions for the very first time, everything from how much you sleep to whom you sleep with. You're dealing with your own fears and foibles and trying to figure out what brings you joy—without taking into consideration the probable reaction of your parents. You're constantly being exposed to things you've never seen before. That's what college was for me: an opportunity to take a hard look at the world and myself.

But arthritis quickly changed all of that. There were restrictions and obligations that other students didn't have. There were appointments with doctors, blood tests, injections, medications and their side effects, major fatigue. Quite honestly, I didn't even pay attention to most of it. I didn't ask questions, I didn't make any effort to be involved in the treatment. A doctor would say, "Amye, we're going to put you on this new medication," and I'd just sort of shrug and say, "Whatever." I didn't know what drugs I was putting into my body and, quite frankly, I didn't care. I was far too deep in denial. My attitude was *Just give me the blasted medicine—give me the silver bullet—and let me get on with my life!*

In hindsight, this was a major mistake. I know today that I should have been much more inquisitive about what was offered to me. I should have asked how it was going to impact the pain, swelling, and destruction going on in my joints; under what conditions was I to take the medications (time of day, with food or not); what side effects and allergic reactions to be aware of; when its effects were to kick in, and how to best contact my doctor if something abnormal were to happen. It is much more productive to be a full partner in your health care. Treat this process with the same passion as you would your favorite hobby, or your boyfriend or girlfriend: with complete interest, attention, and inquisitiveness.

Inevitably, reality began interfering with my fantasy, and it became increasingly difficult to separate Amye the bubbly, ambitious college freshman from Amye the young woman with rheumatoid arthritis. I can recall vividly an instance involving the stairs in our dorm. Negotiating the eight simple steps from the front door to my floor was no small task for me. While all the other girls would be bounding up and down the stairs two at a time, flying along the way young people are wont to do, I would be shuffling slowly, carefully, deliberately.

One leg up . . .

Other leg up . . .

Okay . . . take a breather . . .

Most of the time I was able to keep moving at a pace that didn't attract too much attention, but one day, when my knees were seriously inflamed, I found myself stuck at the bottom of the steps, looking up at the top as if I were looking at the summit of Mount Everest. I held a stack of books in one hand, the railing in the other, and I thought, *How in the world am I going to get up there?*

So I just stood there for a few minutes, saying "Hi" to the dozens of people who cruised right past without so much as a backward glance. Finally, my roommate came by, began bounding up the steps, and suddenly stopped as she hit the landing.

"You all right, Amye?"

"Oh, sure, I'm fine," I responded casually.

She nodded. "All right, see ya later."

Two more strides, and just before she was out of sight, she stopped and turned to face me again. I hadn't moved an inch.

"Are you are sure nothing is wrong? You're moving kind of slow there."

I removed my hand from the rail, tapped the inside of my leg and said, "My knee's bothering me a little. It's an old skiing injury. You go on. I'll be okay."

That seemed to placate her, and soon she was out of sight. Obviously I could have used her help, but I was reluctant to admit the severity of my problem. I was an eighteen-year-old girl with the body of a ninety-year-old. If a part of me was relieved that my roommate hadn't taken pity on me, another part was angry at her lack of sensitivity, but it really had nothing to do with her. She was responding to the information I had given her. That was a valuable lesson. People responded to my words, not my actions. They reacted to the way I portrayed myself, not the way I really was. People close to you might be able to detect the slight limp, the wince when you bend down, the grimace you try to hide, but most people will run right by you. There will be no compassion, no understanding, no assistance. Not because they're insensitive, but because they respond and react to the image you present.

Had I confided in my roommate earlier about how arthritis was affecting my life, it would have been easier to ask for help: "Yeah, my arthritis is really bugging me today and it's painful to do these stairs; can you take my books for me?" Simple and to the point. No sympathy, just empathy . . . and the right kind of help.

I learned early on that it was easy to hide my arthritis with words, because I was a polished speaker. I was friendly and polite. Hey, I was a homecoming queen, so I knew a little something about turning on the charm. This could be especially effective with men, and doubly so when the men were really boys, as is the case when you're in college. Experimenting with the opposite sex is part of the college experience, and like most people I engaged in some lab work. But I was careful not to let a relationship advance to the point of true intimacy. I didn't want anyone to know me that well, because distance was one of my shields.

I tried as hard as I could to keep up with the pace of college life. Everyone else was running around, having fun, going to parties and to movies and dances, and I was lagging behind. Literally. Sometimes I'd be walking across campus with a group of friends and I'd fall behind the pack. They would stop once in a while, turn around and say, "Everything all right back there, Amye?" And I'd say, "Yup, I'm fine. Go ahead and I'll meet you there."

I could have said, "No, it's hard for me to take another step. Can you guys help me?" But I didn't know how to ask for help. As a young person, that's just not part of your training, particularly when you're a college freshman, striving for independence and maturity and a sense of self. You want to do everything on your own— every little thing. I was no different. I yearned to try things, but my body couldn't meet the demands. I wanted to go to parties. I wanted to stand in line at the checkout and buy my own books and carry them to the student lounge to study. I wanted to play tennis. I wanted to run down the hall and burst into someone's room and ask, with breathless anticipation, "Should I wear this dress or this one tonight?" because that's what everyone else was doing. But I couldn't. And the thing about eighteen-year-old girls is if you aren't around, they make other friends.

But no matter your age, when you try to compartmentalize your arthritis, and shut people off from that part of your life, you're going to find yourself very lonely facing this disease on your own. You don't want to be defined by your arthritis, but you can't pretend it doesn't exist. It's a delicate balance, but you have to put arthritis in its appropriate place so that you, and not your disease, is in control of your life.

The only reason I finally came clean with my roommate and told her I had arthritis was because she happened to take a phone message from my doctor's office. Something about more tests and more appointments. Naturally curious, she asked me what was wrong.

"Well," I said, "I have this thing called rheumatoid arthritis."

She scrunched up her nose. An expression of disbelief crossed her face. "Come on! Arthritis is for old people!"

"Yeah, that's what I thought, but I've got it, and sometimes it gives me a bum knee or a sore shoulder, and it can make it kind of hard to get around. But it's really no big deal."

I just passed it off as something insignificant, and she happily accepted my explanation. There was no baring of the soul, no graphic discussion of rheumatoid arthritis and its capacity for devastation. I shrugged it off, and consequently my roommate shrugged it off. That's pretty much the way I got through my entire undergraduate career: by minimizing the disease in the eyes of my friends and classmates.

I wanted to be a typical college student, free of all concerns about health and mortality, but I was having a hard time maintaining the charade. UCSB is a beautiful, sun-drenched waterfront campus. People bike to classes, rather than drive or take a bus, but my hands and knees were so ravaged that I couldn't even think about bicycling. It was all I could do just to walk to class.

My first class each day was at eight A.M., and it was clear across campus from the women's dorm. It's hard for any college student to make an eight-o'clock class, of course. You wake up fifteen minutes before class, throw some water on your face, pull on a T-shirt and a pair of shorts, hop on your bike and fly across campus, and walk in the door just as the professor starts his lecture. For me it was a little more involved than that. I had an eight A.M. biology class that I missed more often than not, primarily because of something known as morning stiffness. Sounds innocent enough, doesn't it? *Morning stiffness.* Well, it can actually be quite restrictive. In arthritis, morning stiffness means the gel in your joints is getting murky, making it extremely difficult to move. It can take hours for the joint to become properly lubricated so that you can walk like anyone else. For me to jump out of bed . . . well, there was just no way. I needed a long, hot shower to start the day. And when I say long, I mean *really* long, like forty-five minutes, maybe even an hour, and as a result I missed a lot of classes. My grades began to suffer. I was always borrowing notes from friends, trying to catch up as best I could. If they asked what was wrong, I'd give them a lame excuse about feeling sick. If I mentioned arthritis, it was always within the context of being something irritating, annoying, but manageable. Certainly I never let on that the disease was now controlling much of my life.

Not that it was easy to hide the severity of my condition. Actually, it took quite a lot of work. Denial is nearly a full-time job, and the stress of trying not to be revealed can take its toll. I remember the first time I attended a college dance after my diagnosis. I had volunteered to take tickets at the door—that seemed not only a great way to check out guys, but it also gave me a chance sit in a chair for a few hours without anyone asking any probing questions. As long as I was sitting down I felt safe and secure; I felt like an equal, because, man, I could talk. In conversation I was anyone's match. But when it came time to stand up and move around, my confidence invariably receded. The more I tried to move, the quieter I became.

Eventually, of course, all the tickets were sold and it was time to move inside. I leaned forward and put all my weight on my elbows so that I wouldn't have to use my hands to stand up. It must have looked odd, because someone asked me if I needed help.

"Nah, just a little stiff from sitting here all evening." *Another day . . . another lie.*

The music was blaring as I entered the room. People were dancing, shouting over the noise, generally just having a good time. As I looked around the room, a wave of anxiety rolled over me: *What if someone asks me to dance?*

This was no small problem. My arthritis was pretty bad at this point. I was in and out of flares, experimenting with various medications, and pushing myself trying to lead what I considered to be a normal life. College kids aren't typically aware of their bodies, at least not in anything other than an aesthetic way, but I was becoming keenly aware of my body, and it terrified me. Parts of me were wracked with pain, but I chose to ignore it. I didn't want to have to focus on what ailed me. That was much too frightening. I wanted to focus on just being a young college student.

Suddenly, someone tapped me on the shoulder.

"Hi, want to dance?"

I had seen this guy when he walked in. In fact, I'd taken his ticket and smiled as he flirted playfully. He seemed nice enough. And he was, I have to admit, pretty cute. So instead of explaining that arthritis was eating away at my knees and hands, or making up some ridiculous story about a hang-gliding accident, I blurted out, "Sure! I'd love to!"

The band was playing a fast song as we walked out on the floor. *How am I going to do this?* But then the answer came to me: I would dance slowly to a fast song, thus not only hiding my affliction, but clearly identifying myself as the coolest chick in the house. You know how there's a coolness associated with doing things slowly, especially when you're young? Well, I took that to an extreme. As the band rocked on, and everyone else jumped around at full throttle, I just sort of swayed back and forth.

Look at me—I'm so cool I can dance slow even when the music is fast.

Placid on the surface, I was utterly turbulent within. Inside I was scared to death that I'd be discovered. Not only that, but my knees were killing me! All that mattered to me, though, was the impression I made on this guy. I fooled him, which was great, but I was also fooling myself, which wasn't so great. I was leading a dual life. I was a young woman in college, being exposed to the wonders of the world, getting educated, growing up, making important decisions for the first time in my life. But behind this manufactured persona, I was wrestling with some formidable demons. However, I wasn't dealing with those demons honestly. I was far too deep in denial to admit their hold on me.

From this struggle I learned something very important, and I would say this to anyone who is coping with any chronic illness: Denial is a terrible and powerful thing that one day will explode inside you, sending shock waves of regret, fear, and pain throughout your body and mind. You'll question everything you've done, everything that has led you to this point, and you'll probably feel helpless and stupid. When you finally realize that you've been in denial, you may wonder what other aspects of your life denial has clouded. But try not to be too hard on yourself. The lessons of denial have a way of showing you how you handle crises and challenges. Still, it's better to confront the disease early on your own terms, before it confronts you.

I was confronted again, in rather embarrassing fashion, after what should have been a harmless afternoon of sunbathing. This was Southern California, so kids often wore bathing suits to classes, or at least bathing suits under their clothes, so that they'd be ready on a moment's notice to take advantage of the sunny weather. It wasn't at all unusual to go straight from the classroom to the beach or the tennis courts. One afternoon, my girlfriends and I were sitting on the lawn in front of our dorm, sunning ourselves. This was a mistake. Chronic fatigue is a major component of arthritis. You're always tossing and turning in the middle of the night, waking abruptly and in pain because you've rolled over onto a particularly sensitive joint. I was getting by on about five or six hours of sleep a night at this time, and I should have known better than to lie down in the sun on a hot afternoon. But I did it anyway. We were all talking, having a good time, and the next thing I knew it was three hours later. I lifted my head up off my blanket to discover that the sun was now low in the sky and I was all alone. The ocean breeze was picking up, and I was cold and disoriented.

Where did everybody go?

I slowly tried to pull myself into a sitting position, but found to my dismay that I could barely move. Three hours in the breeze, lying on hard ground, had stiffened my joints nearly to the point of immobility.

Thanks, girlfriends! How am I going to get up?

So I stayed there for a while, trying to figure out a reasonable solution for my dilemma. If I yelled for help, I'd look like a cripple. If I tried to stand up, I'd *really* look like a cripple. Either way, I'd be presenting an image I considered unacceptable and distasteful.

Eventually I managed to roll over and sit up, but that was about as far as I could go. When a pleasant-looking young fellow walked by, I shouted to get his attention, but I tried to do so in a calm, controlled way, so that my voice would betray neither the anger nor fear I was experiencing.

"Hey, you mind giving me hand?" I said.

He smiled, yelled "No problem," and walked right over.

"Sorry," I explained. "I went skiing last week and hurt my knee, and it gets real stiff on me sometimes."

Accepting my explanation implicitly, he extended a hand and pulled me to my feet. I clenched my teeth so as not to yell, thanked him for his help, and went inside. As I got closer to my dorm, I could see my girlfriends standing in the window of my bedroom, laughing hysterically. It turned out this was their idea of a joke! But it had nothing to do with my arthritis. No, they just wanted to see how I'd react when I woke up alone.

"Man, Amye, you were snoring like a banshee," one of them said with a laugh. "We tried to wake you up, but you were half dead."

The anger dissipated quickly. I was actually honored that they would play a joke on me and not think I would get upset. It was a gesture of friendship, nothing more or less. At the same time I was scared to death that they would discover the truth: that my arthritis was so pronounced that I could barely stand up. But even when they saw this guy lifting me to my feet, they didn't get it. My secret was safe.

I was into so much denial that I refused to become educated about arthritis. Consequently, when my symptoms got worse or flared, I would panic. When you hear a fire alarm go off in your office or dorm, you know exactly what to do, because you've been instructed. That fire alarm was going off in my body regularly, but because I didn't *choose* to find out what to do, it was a natural instinct just to panic.

I remember one time, after I was on aspirin therapy for about four months, I experienced a terrible ringing sensation in my ears—*Eeeeeeehhhhhhhh*—as if a mosquito had burrowed inside my head. It freaked me out! For a while I was using Q-tips to try to dig it out. But when that didn't work I called my doctor in tears. He calmly explained that the aspirin therapy had probably given me a nasty case of tinnitus. No one had told me that tinnitus is a side effect of aspirin therapy, and I hadn't asked.

That's one of the reasons I'm such an arthritis health advocate today: I learned the hard way that your own inactions can alter the course of your disease. It's important to be aware of the benefits and consequences of your medications, and to be a partner in your own treatment. I never knew when I was supposed to call the doctor, when it was entirely appropriate, even necessary. I was always afraid someone would accuse me of crying wolf. But if you don't ask, you'll never know. And there is powerful strength in knowing what you're up against.

So I wandered aimlessly through my treatment, never asking enough questions, never doing enough research or homework. I woke each morning hoping I'd feel well enough to go to class, and if I did, I pretty much put arthritis out of my mind for the day.

As a young person, the first thing you want to do, or feel you should do, in times of crisis, is call your parents. But I was hesitant to do that because I was trying to be an adult. In fact, even though they were closer to me than anyone else on the planet, my parents were often the last to know when I had flares or other problems related to arthritis. As a result, they didn't understand just how far the disease had progressed. Once, during a holiday meal, my reticence led to an illuminating confrontation.

It was traditional in my home for the women to clean up after meals. But on this night I was feeling particularly weak. When dinner was over, my mom and my sister got up and began clearing the table, but I just slumped down in my seat.

"Come on, Amye," Mom said. "Time to do the dishes."

Now, I knew it was time to do the dishes, but I just couldn't. My knees ached, my knuckles were swollen. My whole body felt feverish. I didn't say anything. I just let Mom and J work around me. A few minutes later my mother emerged from the kitchen. "Are you going to sit there all night?"

"I can't get up, Mom."

She stared at me blankly. "What do you mean you can't get up?"

My family knew about my arthritis, but you see, it's more complicated than that. Arthritis is not always obvious, and when you're going to great lengths to hide it, as I was, people aren't always quick to acknowledge when you finally reveal a flare.

"I hurt too much, Mom," I said. "It's my arthritis."

"Yeah, okay," she said calmly. "When you're ready to help with the dishes, let us know."

The look on my mother's face was that parental look—*You're lying, you're just being lazy*—and then she turned and walked away.

I've learned a lot of lessons since then. I've learned that sometimes you have to be extremely graphic in the way you describe what you're feeling: *"It's like someone is sticking razor blades into my kneecaps!"* You have to be convincing. That's hard, I know, because you don't want to seem weak. You don't want to be a burden. Sometimes, though, a good, bloody description of your pain is the only way to get the point across. In families, of course, it's a bit more complicated, because family members often don't listen to one another. There's so much history, so many conflicting emotions. I was a good student and never caused my parents any trouble while growing up. Undeniably, though, I was a strong-willed, rambunctious kid who didn't mind a good argument now and then. I'm sure there were times in the early years after my diagnosis when my parents thought I was just trying to get away with something, just as I had as a child. It's taken years for my family to fully understand what it means to have arthritis. They are my biggest advocates now, my most loyal supporters, but it was a long, slow process of discovery and communication. In fact, it was about seven or eight years after my diagnosis before they finally got the point. I don't blame them. Because of denial, it took almost that long for me to comprehend it.

Arthritis is a tease. It changes you gradually, imperceptibly at first. Then it ebbs and flows. The gray cloud moves in, ruins your life for a while, then it moves out. But it always comes back. Without appropriate treatment, help, and psychosocial support, over time, the overcast days outnumber the clear days, until you wake up one morning and realize you can't recall the last time you saw the sun.

5

Wings of Desire

There is fear, and then there is *fear*. The first envelops you slowly, fills you with dread and anxiety over the course of weeks, months, even years. It's worry and anger mixed together and brought to a steady boil. That's what happens when you are diagnosed with rheumatoid arthritis: the anticipation of an erosion of your lifestyle sucks the strength right out of you and makes it easier for the disease to take root.

The second type of fear is more palpable, immediate. It's the kind you experience when someone puts a gun to your head, or the brakes on your car fail. Or, perhaps, when you're careening through a raging midwestern snowstorm in an eight-seat turboprop.

After graduating from college, I had gone home for a few months. I had my heart set on graduate school, but I knew I'd need some time to get my arthritis under control. Before long, though, I was eager to get out of town, to resume my academic and personal education. Rather than pursue a master's in business administration in California, which would have been the sensible thing to do, given my reliance on doctors and family and friends, I opted for Purdue University, located in West Lafayette, Indiana.

Purdue was captivating for a couple of reasons. First of all, my speech instructor in high school had been a graduate of Purdue, and the memory of him describing a beautiful campus and a friendly, accommodating faculty had stayed with me over the years; he had painted such a pretty picture. I admired this teacher and I respected his opinion, so Purdue was always high on my list of potential graduate schools. Second, when I began investigating MBA programs, I discovered that they are typically rote—there's an emphasis on how to run a business, how to manage an organization, that sort of thing. I was more interested in the personal aspect of business. Purdue, at the time, had one of two MBA programs in the country that focused heavily on industrial relations, which was exactly what I wanted. The other program was at Columbia University in New York. Columbia, I determined, was just too far from home and too cold. Purdue would be more hospitable, or so I thought. Little did I know that West Lafayette, Indiana, while a lovely enough place in the spring and summer, is practically arctic in the winter months. It's cold, flat, and windy; storms regularly barrel across the midwestern plains and drop several feet of snow on unsuspecting California transplants just for laughs.

At my going-away party in Bakersfield, some of my friends gave me a little miniature pair of snowshoes. "You'll need these at Purdue," they said.

I laughed. "How cute! Thanks so much. But it's really not that bad there."

I expected a few friendly flakes now and then, just enough to give the whole experience a sense of adventure. On some level, I sought an element of danger—that was all part of striving for independence while afflicted with a disease that threatened to leave me housebound. Purdue seemed like a reasonable compromise: it

was far from home, but not as far from home as New York; the climate was harsh, but not so harsh that I'd be unable to survive, even
with arthritis; most important of all, it offered one of the best MBA
programs in the nation for someone interested in industrial relations. Whatever the environment was, I'd learn how to deal with it.

All that sounded logical enough from the safety and security of
Bakersfield. Ten thousand feet in the air, bouncing through a bliz-
zard in a plane that looked like something Lindbergh might have
flown, my reasoning suddenly seemed flawed.

What is this? Alaska? I'm going to die before I take my first class!

The trip had begun innocuously enough, with a smooth flight on
a jumbo jet from L.A. to Chicago. But in Chicago I boarded a small
commuter plane, and from there the journey took a decidedly
frightful turn. We were getting tossed all over the sky. Luggage was
falling, passengers were bouncing high out of their seats and
smacking their heads on the ceiling. At one point we hit a particularly rough patch of air and quickly dropped about five hundred
feet. My heart jumped into my throat, and I closed my eyes and
began to pray.

*Please, God . . . just get me on the ground and I'll take a bus right back
to California.*

I admonished myself for being so naive. You see, I hadn't even
taken a trip to Purdue to look at the campus. I had stubbornly and
blindly made a decision to attend the school, and they had made a
decision to accept me based solely on the strength of my undergraduate academic record, recommendations, and test scores.
When I received my acceptance letter, I was quite proud of the fact
that they had demonstrated such a leap of faith. Now I was kicking
myself for being so impetuous.

*I can't believe how stupid I am! Look at all this snow! How am I going
to get around? I don't know how to drive in this stuff. Heck, I don't even
know how to walk in it! I have arthritis, for God's sake! What if I fall
down? I'll freeze to death, and they'll never find me.*

Please! Turn this plane around! I WANT TO GO HOME!!

We landed at the smallest airport I'd ever seen. I climbed down a rickety set of steps and picked up my bags, which had been tossed out onto the tarmac. With the wind howling and the snow sticking to my face, I looked around at the desolate landscape and said, to no one in particular, "What have I gotten myself into?"

I walked to a little brick building—the lone terminal—and started searching my pockets for some change so that I could call a cab. Inside, though, was a stately gentleman who was clearly waiting for someone. Our eyes met, he smiled warmly, and approached with his hand extended.

"Amye?"

I recognized the voice instantly. It belonged to Purdue's dean of students. We had talked several times on the phone, and I had told him when I'd be arriving. But I had no idea he would be meeting me at the airport. At that moment, he might as well have been Santa Claus to me.

"How was the trip?" he asked.

I bit my tongue. "Oh, fine." It was time to start being brave.

"Yeah? Well, if it's any consolation, you should know that this is about as bad as the weather gets." He gestured toward the front door. "Come on, let me show you your new home."

Within a few weeks of my arrival at Purdue, I had slipped comfortably back into a state of denial. It didn't take long for me to realize that the MBA program's reputation was well deserved. It was a rigorous, intensely competitive, two-year program. Unlike the undergraduate population at UCSB, the MBA students at Purdue not only attended all of their classes but also usually showed up ahead of time. People paid attention. They took copious notes. They asked a lot of questions. They debated with their professors and their fellow students. If you missed something, you were responsible for making up the work, and very few students seemed at ease with the notion of sharing notes: It was, quite literally, every man for himself.

For me, this was at once exhilarating and terrifying. The young adult was invigorated by the need for independence; the arthritis victim found it intimidating. Complicating matters was my quandary over how much to divulge: *Whom do I tell . . . and how do I tell them?* I didn't want anyone to think less of me because of my arthritis; and yet, if a problem arose because of my arthritis—if I suddenly flared—I would need an ally. The solution was to handle it on a case-by-case basis. If one of my friends saw I was having difficulty and asked, "What's wrong?" I would tell her. I was more direct than I had been in college, more clear about the nature of the disease and the fact that I might need some help. As usual, most people were perplexed by the idea of a twenty-two-year-old with arthritis, but a few good souls took it in stride and offered to assist in any way possible.

The shock of my first day in West Lafayette proved to be less of an omen than I had feared. Thanks to a series of underground tunnels connecting the graduate dorms to Krannert Graduate School, where I took most of my classes, I rarely had to deal with the elements. The tunnels were nicely lit and clean, and you could actually roll right out of bed, walk to an elevator, take the elevator to the tunnels, and then walk all the way to your classes without seeing a single snowflake, even in the middle of January. There were two or three of us from the West Coast in the MBA program, and we all lived in the graduate dorm. We used to taunt the other grad students who lived off campus. We'd show up in shorts and sandals and Hawaiian-print T-shirts, while they'd be peeling off layers of wet fleece and down after having trudged through the snow.

In focusing so intensely on my studies, I neglected my health. When old, familiar aches and twinges began to appear, I simply ignored them. I was far too busy working hard, applying myself, and getting established as a serious student to leave any room in my life for rheumatoid arthritis. But as the pain spread and intensified, I was compelled to deal with it. First, I formed a relationship with a new doctor—not a rheumatologist, mind you, but an orthopedic surgeon who spent most of his time tending to broken bones and sprained ligaments. Before long I was getting weekly injections of immunosuppresive drugs and taking all kinds of anti-inflammatory medications to no avail. I'd been down this slippery slope before. But I was determined to beat the disease on my own terms. As the semester wore on, I found myself hurting all over. My hands, knees, neck, and feet were all inflamed at the same time. The disease was moving slowly but deliberately, eating my body one joint at a time.

You learn a lot about yourself in a hypercompetitive environment. You find out not only how much you like to win, but also how tough you are, and how compassionate you are. You learn valuable lessons that pertain to life as well as the classroom and the boardroom. Unfortunately, this is not necessarily the best environment for someone with a chronic illness. Like most of my classmates, I stayed up studying until twelve or one each night. Unlike my classmates, I didn't have the ability to simply pop out of bed in the morning and run to class. The morning stiffness that had made one-hour showers a mandatory part of my morning ritual in college had returned with a vengeance in graduate school. Now I would wake up, gobble a handful of pills, take a long, hot shower, crawl back under the covers for an hour or so while the pills went to work, and if they worked, I'd get dressed and go to class. Sleep became an elusive prize, so deep and relentless was the throbbing in my joints. I'd wake at four in the morning, my knees on fire, my head pounding. There were times when I wished I could have amputated my own legs, just to be rid of the searing pain. I seemed always to be in the grips of the worst case of the flu imaginable. I was feverish, sore, exhausted. I couldn't take proper care of myself, couldn't brush my teeth or comb my hair. I wasn't eating right.

Worse, I had no one with whom I could share this information, not in any substantive way. I had a deal with my parents: I'd call once a week just to let them know how I was doing, but I tried very hard not to share my misery with them, for I knew they would only panic, and there was nothing they could do from fifteen hundred miles away. But eventually, I informed my parents of my condition, and they were of course worried.

"Dad, I'm hurting all the time now," I said during one of our phone conversations. "I'm taking all the medication they're prescribing, and nothing seems to be working. I'm crying myself to sleep every night."

He was silent on the other end, and in his silence I heard fatherly concern. After a few moments he responded. "Amye . . . honey?"

"Yeah, Dad?"

"I think you need to go to the hospital."

My first reaction was *No way!* Going to the hospital in graduate school means not going to classes, and missing classes means falling behind, and falling behind means making up work, and . . . well, a proud, competitive woman in a competitive environment just doesn't acquiesce that easily. So I balked. Stubbornly refusing to seek help, I kept going to class and studying late into the night.

I am stronger than this disease, and I will not let it get the best of me!

Wrong again. I flared to an unprecedented degree a few nights later. The pain rolled over me like a tidal wave, knocking me to the ground and slapping the belligerence right out of me. It was like nothing I had experienced in all of my previous battles with arthritis. The doctor took one look at me and immediately suggested admitting me to PUSH (Purdue University Student Hospital). Even in my weakened and disoriented state, I tried to decline the invitation.

"Can't miss classes," I said. "I'll fall behind."

He twisted his face into a look of bemusement. I'm not sure whether he found my spunk entertaining or infuriating.

"Look, Amye," he said. "You can barely walk. You're going to have to forget about school for a little while. Let's get you squared away physically, find out what's wrong, and then we can deal with the other stuff later."

In retrospect, I can see he was being the voice of reason, and I'm grateful for that. He really didn't prescribe anything different, but he knew I needed to get off my feet. So he ordered complete bed rest. Interestingly, though, something about that prescription—*bed rest*—indicated to me that I wasn't actually all that sick. I remember lying in my hospital bed after a day or two thinking *I could do this in my dorm room. I could get my books, relax, read, take notes, and I'd be just fine.*

"Hey, Doc. How about a change of venue?" I suggested.

"Such as?"

"My dorm."

"Absolutely not! You need complete bed rest. That means no telephone, no reading, no studying . . . nothing!"

He was right, of course. I was very sick. When my blood work came back from the lab I was informed that my electrolytes were completely out of kilter and my sedimentation rate, which reflects the amount of inflammation in your system, was huge. Now, years later, I know how to recognize and identify a massive flare in its early stages. Back then I was too inexperienced, too young, too stubborn.

While everyone at PUSH was nice enough, they simply gave me pain medication and told me to rest. In fact, that was the very first time I had ever received any pain medication, and while it proved to be effective enough, it also put me in something close to a vegetative state. Pain medication, for me, is one giant sleeping pill. I can't think straight when I'm taking painkillers of any kind; I can barely talk. As for schoolwork? Forget about it. I spent the better part of the next three weeks riding a cloud. I slept fifteen, eighteen hours a day.

Today, obviously, with managed-care health insurance, it's hard to imagine being hospitalized for twenty-one days when the full extent of your treatment is bed rest. But this was a long time ago, and it was a student hospital. I was there under my student health plan.

Moreover, I was in a unique position: they couldn't just send me back to the dorm because I could barely walk or get myself dressed or feed myself. My protestations to the contrary notwithstanding, I was incapable of caring for myself in the graduate dorm, and the doctors, to their credit, knew this.

Discharging me would have been dangerous and irresponsible. I wasn't even eating, which was a remarkable thing in itself since I really love food. I love everything about it—the preparation, the chemistry, the creativity, the social aspects of a good dining experience. *Everything.* It was during this period of crisis that I began to see how the body and mind react to pain, and how I specifically react. Everybody has a unique way of dealing with discomfort, with stress. When I hurt, I don't eat. It's not a control issue for me, although that is the case with some people, especially women, who suffer from chronic illness. In the days and weeks leading up to my hospitalization, I was just too exhausted to eat. I didn't care about food, I didn't like the way it looked or smelled or tasted. I've had this unpleasant experience numerous times over the years. When I'm in severe pain, my taste buds seem to fail. All my senses are off. So dining, which is normally such a delightful experience, becomes an exercise, a chore, and I lose interest. Later, when I was recovering from going through numerous joint-replacement surgeries, and I'd be hospitalized for weeks at a time, my mother would do her best to get me to eat by preparing my favorite foods and bringing them to the hospital, in the hope that my senses would respond to the smells and tastes they knew best. Sometimes it worked, sometimes it didn't, but it's a strategy I heartily endorse. If you're having an arthritis flare or if you're hospitalized, it's particularly important to maintain your strength, and one of the ways you do that is by eating nutritious foods. Make foods you really enjoy, or have someone else make them for you. Do whatever you can to stimulate your taste buds and fuel your immune system.

During the final week of my hospitalization at PUSH, at a time when I was trying to kick the painkillers and starting to feel a bit better about myself, I received a sobering visit from one of my professors. By this time I was getting precious few visitors. My friends and classmates had come by frequently in the first week, but they had their own lives to attend to, their own classes to take. The reality of the situation was that people began to forget about me. I was out of the dorm, out of the classroom, out of the picture, out of the loop. I had become a ghost. That's why it was such a surprise to see my statistics professor standing in the doorway one morning. I wasn't especially fond of him or his course. I'm a people person by nature and took statistics only because it was a requirement of my MBA program. It was a large class and I wasn't well known, at least not up to that point. I'd been admitted to the hospital rather suddenly and therefore hadn't had an opportunity to meet with each of my professors to discuss my impending absence; I never told any of them, "Sorry, but I have rheumatoid arthritis and I can't hold a pen, so I'm going to be in the hospital for a while. Hope you understand." Uh-uh. There was nothing like that. I just vanished. *Poof!*

At some point the dean of students had contacted my professors and alerted them to my condition. But that still didn't explain why my statistics professor was in my room. We had no relationship; of all my teachers, he would have been the last one I expected to visit.

"Amye, how are you?" he asked.

I pulled myself up in bed and tried to manage a smile. "Well, I've been better."

He nodded. "What's the prognosis?"

I wasn't quite sure how to answer. Obviously he knew I was sick— I was in a hospital bed and hadn't been in his class for nearly three weeks, but I wasn't sure whether he knew the details behind my hospitalization. Not wanting him to think less of me, I carefully avoided use of the dreaded *D* word—*disease*—and explained as succinctly as possible that I had something called rheumatoid arthritis. "Usually it's no big deal," I lied, "but sometimes it really causes me some grief." I chuckled slightly. "Like now."

I was trying to convince my professor that my affliction was relatively benign, but I wasn't doing a very good job of it. I could tell by the look on his face that he was thinking, *I'm standing in front of a very sick girl in a hospital bed, and she's telling me everything's okay. Hmmmmm. What's wrong with this picture?*

"You've been in the hospital for quite a while now," he said solemnly. "Usually, when a person has been in the hospital this long, it's very serious. I've talked to the dean, and as I understand it, you're pretty sick."

With a feeble wave of my hand, I dismissed his concern entirely. "No, no, no. Not me. As soon as they get my medication straightened out, I'll be good as new." I forced a smile and tried to change the subject. "So, how's class, anyway?"

My professor looked down at his feet and thought deeply before speaking. "You know, Amye," he began, "I'm aware of how hard you've been working, and I think that's great. I really do. But you have to understand, this is a very competitive school, and a very competitive class. If for some reason you're unable to complete your course work . . . well, maybe it's not the best time for you to be in graduate school."

My jaw dropped open. I looked at him and thought, *You've already passed judgment on me. You've declared me dead! How dare you?!* My blood began to boil. I think this was the very first time in my life that I tried to channel all the anger and frustration—the byproducts of rheumatoid arthritis—into something useful. I wasn't going to shout at him; rather, I directed all my energy into being deliberate, forceful, determined. It was almost as if I could feel the molecules coming together in my body, pushing the words from my stomach into my mouth.

"Look, Professor, I'm not stupid. Rheumatoid arthritis does not affect my mind. I am in pain right now, and it's true that the pain medication makes me sleepy and I haven't been able to attend your class. But the pain will subside. I'm already feeling better."

He rubbed his chin with his hand, removed his glasses, and gave me a hard look. "I don't know . . ."

"I want to continue in your class," I said. "All I ask from you and my friends is some assistance so that I can get the proper notes. I can't physically get to class right now, but that won't last much longer. In the meantime, I can do my studying in the hospital and in my dorm room; I can take all the tests, complete all the papers. We can have conversations about the course material over the phone, if you'd like. You set the parameters, and I'll abide by them. Just don't quit on me. Please."

We went back and forth like this for a while, with him throwing up obstacles and me hammering away at them. Eventually, he relented.

"Amye, I admire your determination," he said. "You have a lot of studying to do; you've fallen far behind your classmates. But if you really think you can catch up . . ."

"I can," I interrupted. "Just watch me."

"Do you know how much longer you're going to be in the hospital?"

"No, but I'll talk to the doctor this afternoon and get a better idea. And then I'll let you know." I was willing to say anything to save my bony little tush. The truth was, I didn't know whether I could make up the work, and I didn't know how my doctor would react when I told him I planned to start studying—immediately— whether he liked it or not. No one else was going to act as my advocate, so I had to accept the role myself. Before the week was out, I'd have plenty of practice.

When my statistics professor left, I felt almost euphoric. The victory was sweet. I remember thinking, *How strange. I'm ecstatic because I'm being allowed to remain in a class that bores me to tears, taught by a professor I don't understand.* Such is the nature of chronic illness: you find joy in the oddest of circumstances.

Four hours later, another of my professors walked into my room, and I immediately sensed that he and my statistics professor had shared notes.

"I got a call from the dean of students and I just wanted to see how you're doing," he said. The smile faded from his face and his brow furrowed. "How are you doing?"

Hmmmmm. Let's see. What to say? Evasiveness didn't work all that well this morning, so let's try plain old lying.

"I'm doing great!" I said. "When I first got here I was in pretty rough shape, but now I'm feeling fine."

"What is it you have?"

"Rheumatoid arthritis, and it's completely controlled by medication. For some reason my medication got all screwed up and I needed some bed rest so they could monitor my blood levels and boost my strength. But it's all under control now. I'll be getting out soon—maybe even today!"

I could almost feel my nose growing. Not only that, but this professor was no fool. He, too, saw the discrepancy between the person in front of him and the image she was trying to present.

"I was told you couldn't even walk," he said. "That sounds pretty bad. I have to be honest, Amye. I'm concerned about you and I'm concerned about your ability to successfully complete this class. Maybe you need to take some time off and come back next semester."

Ahhhh . . . here we go again. Another wolf in a different type of clothing. He's feigning concern, when what he really wants is not to have to deal with me or my disability.

Once again I could feel the molecules coming together, giving me strength. This time, however, I opted for a gentler approach, one that included a heavy dose of flattery. "What I would really like is to stay in this class," I said. "I *love* this class. I'm getting so much out of it."

More shaking of the head, more hand wringing. "I don't know, Amye. You've missed so much already."

All right, pal. You want me to be a brown nose? Then that's what I'll be.

"Professor, you are a wonderful teacher and I have learned so much in your class. *(Yech!)* Don't take that away from me. My friends will help me get notes and I'll make up all of the work. Believe me, you won't be disappointed."

He let out a heavy sigh. *Got him!*

"All right, then. It's against my better judgment, but we'll give it a shot." He hesitated, looked around the room, and added, "Good luck."

So it went for the rest of the week. Every one of my professors paid a visit, ostensibly to see how I was doing, but really to encourage me to quit school. Each time I endured a painful negotiating session, and each time I emerged triumphant. What an incredible feeling! To be bedridden, and yet still have the power to control my own destiny, my own fate, simply by using the right words. I don't mean to be hyperbolic, but as I saw it, nothing less than my life was at stake. Repeating any of those courses would have been disastrous at that time. My goal of completing graduate school on schedule would have been lost; more important, each withdrawal, each *incomplete* on my transcript would have represented a major victory for this damnable disease. I wasn't about to let that happen.

Within a week I was released from the hospital and returned to my dorm room. With the assistance of a handful of friends I made up the work I had missed and successfully completed every course. Now, when I say "successfully," I mean B's and C's. Ordinarily, these were not good grades for me. I had always been an A student. Under the circumstances, though, I considered five grades of C or better to be quite an accomplishment. Along the way I had learned something valuable, something I wasn't taught in any of my classes. I learned that in order to change opinions and change people's minds, you have to understand their perceptions and let them know that what they see may not be accurate. And you have to do it in an authoritative way, so it's clear that you are in control. You are the one who knows your disease. They don't know anything about it. Therefore, you have to explain to your audience what it is you have, how it does and does not affect you, and how you can work together to fight it. This is true in the workplace, school, and in relationships.

My second year at Purdue was less eventful. Arthritis is a roller-coaster ride of a disease, and I was in a smooth period through much of my second year. My grades improved and I had a better social life, but arthritis was never far from my mind. Whenever I slipped into denial, or tried to convince myself I had been miraculously cured, the disease would make its presence known. Sometimes subtly, sometimes vividly.

I lived off campus that year, and once, while waiting for a bus, my friend Patty suggested we make snow angels in the newly fallen powder.

"Snow angels?" I said. Hey, I was from California. Where I come from, snow angels are the dealers who work the corners of some of L.A.'s less desirable neighborhoods.

"Sure," Patty said. "Watch. It's easy."

She held her arms wide, parallel to the ground, and fell backward into the snow. *Whump!* After landing, she began flapping her arms and legs, as if she were doing jumping jacks in the snow. When she stood up, the impression left behind did indeed look like an angel with gorgeous, white wings.

"Try it," Patty said.

"Okay." I plopped into the snow ever so gingerly, thinking, *Is this going to hurt? And how will I get up?*

Well, it didn't hurt at all, and Patty was there to help me up, but I couldn't move my arms very well. My coat was too bulky, the snow too heavy, my joints too weak. So, after I stood, Patty and I turned to examine my snow angel. And there it was—an angel with clipped wings.

We made a joke about Amye's pathetic angel, but inside I was saddened, because that snow angel represented what I was losing: the ability to soar . . . to fly . . .*to be free.*

6

Going It Alone

By the time I graduated from Purdue, I felt like I was on top of the world, like there was nothing I couldn't accomplish if I put my mind to it. The university, to its credit, had instilled this feeling in me, and in all of its students. In the field of industrial relations, there weren't many programs better than Purdue's, so my newly minted MBA carried a significant amount of weight, and I carried it proudly, confidently.

One of the first things I did during my job hunt was write a letter to a woman named Frances Lear, who at that time was married to Norman Lear, a very successful television producer whose credits included the groundbreaking hit *All in the Family*. Frances was a dynamic, talented woman in her own right who ran a top-notch executive recruitment firm in Century City, California, and occasionally wrote articles for business magazines and other publications. It was after reading one of these articles, about women in the workplace, that I felt compelled to write her—she seemed like such a smart, gutsy lady that I just couldn't resist trying to make contact. My raging confidence notwithstanding, I fully expected the letter (and the accompanying resume) to go straight into that repository of all unsolicited correspondence, the circular file, but lo and behold, a few weeks later, I got a response. She said she was impressed by my credentials and that, if I was ever in Los Angeles, I should give her a call.

Wow! This was almost too good to be true. What Frances didn't know was that I had every intention of going to L.A., and not just to visit. Although I had received job offers from employers in the Midwest and Northeast, none was enticing enough to convince me that life wouldn't be easier, and better, in Southern California. Quite frankly, I'd seen enough snow and ice to last a lifetime.

I called Frances as soon as I got home, and we quickly arranged an interview. I remember wearing a green pantsuit and carrying a purse and a briefcase. When I got to the office I was disappointed to learn that Frances had been called away on an emergency, so I would be meeting with her partner, Archie Purvis. When Archie and I sat down, I thought, *Well, this will be short.* I was fresh out of graduate school, sitting in a big, beautiful office, in a big, beautiful building, and my contact, the woman who had expressed interest in me, was nowhere to be found. I assumed, incorrectly as it turned out, that Mr. Purvis was merely being polite by stepping in for his partner. We wound up chatting for nearly three hours, at the end of which he said, "Well, young lady, I have two things to say."

I nodded eagerly.

"One . . . lose the purse."

"Lose the purse?" I had no idea what he was talking about.

"Uh-huh. You present very well, but never walk into an interview carrying a purse *and* a briefcase. It looks . . . cumbersome."

"Okay," I said. "What else?" I braced myself for more criticism.

"Two . . . we don't normally represent people in entry-level positions . . ."

Here it comes, the kiss-off . . .

"But in your case, we're going to make an exception. We'd like to represent you."

For a second I felt numb. I could barely speak.

"Really?"

He smiled. "Really. We work with all the top companies in Los Angeles, and we'll be happy to talk with them on your behalf. If we hear of an opening, we'll give you a buzz."

Archie extended his hand to close the deal, and as we shook, another thought came to mind. "How am I going to pay for this?" I said.

Archie frowned, as if to say, *Don't worry.* "Look, we believe in you. Frances liked you on paper, and I like you in person. You actually are what you represent yourself to be on your resume, and believe me, that's rare."

I didn't doubt that, because, in reality, I wasn't exactly the person on my resume, either. In truth, I was a young woman with a serious, debilitating case of rheumatoid arthritis, a woman in serious denial about her condition. Only when the illness flared so badly that I was nearly incapacitated did I acknowledge its presence. In times of remission, I ignored it, pretended it didn't exist. Like everyone else, I embraced the notion that arthritis was "for old people." And I wasn't old.

Archie and Frances came through for me with impressive speed and efficiency. I began having interviews within just a few days, and in a matter of weeks I had my first job, a midlevel management position with a telecommunications company. I moved to Marina del Rey, California, and got myself a nice waterfront apartment. Why Marina del Rey? Because that's where all the pretty people lived. I thought, *Hey, I'm a pretty person, too. I should live there!* I was making a good salary, had a nice car, and when I went to sleep at night I could hear the sound of the sailboats rocking in the water and the clanging of their bells in the breeze. On good nights—and there were quite a few of them—I couldn't help but think of how lucky I was.

My arthritis was there, always lurking in the background, but I really wasn't interested in it. I wasn't paying attention to it. Marina del Rey was all about a certain lifestyle and attitude, and I found myself easily seduced by it. If you were an attractive woman in Marina del Rey, you could have most anything you wanted. I started meeting a lot of men and went out on a lot of dates, but I often behaved oddly. I'd go out to dinner, or to a movie, and sometimes I'd be willing to go on a second date, maybe even a third. Invariably, though, the moment I felt the relationship growing intimate, I'd cut it off. It dawned on me after a while that the reason I was withdrawing had nothing to do with fear of commitment, or the search for the perfect guy, but simply fear of rejection—more to the point, fear of getting caught, of being discovered. Even though it was not very visible during my early months in Marina del Rey, I was afraid someone would find out about my arthritis. I'd been given a chance to reinvent myself as a healthy, active woman, someone who didn't have arthritis or any other disability, and I was loath to reveal the truth. As a result, I kept most people, especially most men, at a safe and comfortable distance.

That all changed one afternoon when I was standing on my balcony, looking out at the boats docked below. On one of the boats was a pleasant-looking gentleman, and as soon as our eyes met, he waved and smiled.

"You new here?" he shouted.

"Uh-huh."

"Come on down and have a drink with us."

As he spoke, another man appeared on the deck of the boat. He, too, smiled and waved.

I don't know why, but something told me they were decent people and that I had nothing to fear. Time and circumstance would support that initial impression, because these two men, Ron and Danny, were not only neighbors in my apartment complex, but two of the most wonderful people I have ever had the privilege to know. In fact, they've been like brothers to me for many years. They were as different as night and day, and I was quite different from them, but somehow we became like family, and they became my support system. They looked out for me and took care of me, just as they would a younger sister, and in turn I treated them like brothers, which is to say I admired them, worried about them, and gave them endless grief about the women in their lives. It's a measure of the depth of our friendship that eventually I told Ron and Danny all about my arthritis. They were the first two people in Marina del Rey to learn of my hidden disability, and, predictably, their first reaction was disbelief.

"Come on," Ron said. "You're too young to have arthritis."

"Yeah, I know, but I have it anyway. There are times when it's hard to function, times when I can barely walk. But most of the time I'm all right. I just want you guys to know."

And that was that. I presented the truth matter-of-factly, and they accepted it with a shrug. Not because they didn't believe me, and certainly not because they didn't care. Like everyone else with whom I'd shared this secret over the years, they found the picture to be inconsistent with the information, and therefore difficult to comprehend. So we let it go.

We established routines that made life enormously enjoyable, like Tuesday night at the movies. First it was just the three of us. Then we were joined by three more people . . . and three more. Pretty soon we had groups of twelve, fifteen people going to the movies every Tuesday evening after work. Before long the threesome of Ron, Danny, and Amye became the focal point of the social scene at our apartment complex. We threw parties for two hundred people. We had a St. Patrick's Day party with kegs of green beer, and a May Day party with mountains of flowers, and along the way these two men became incredibly protective of me and my condition. They saw me enough to get glimpses into the world of rheumatoid arthritis, and they responded with support and sympathy, but never pity. If we were out in a park, and I was having trouble walking, they would instinctively, and silently, slow down. If we went to the movies, they'd drop me off at the door before parking. They didn't make a big deal out of it; they just did it. I'd never experienced anything like this before—a real *friendship* with a man, and now two men, to boot. These two men became two of my closest, most intimate friends; they were my family away from home. They knew all my deepest, darkest secrets, and I knew theirs. It's very hard to explain how something like this develops. We wanted to have fun—that was the foundation for our friendship—but we also wanted, and needed, something more. Support . . . companionship . . . love.

At times it seemed like a movie or a sitcom. We'd be up late at night on weekends, talking until we couldn't keep our eyes open, and then we'd fall asleep in the same bed, like trusting siblings. And when we'd wake up in the morning, someone would already be making breakfast. It was an unwritten rule: *First one up cooks the eggs.* It was that kind of familial support that kept me going at a time when I was really trying very hard to pretend I was someone else. Ron and Danny knew me to the core, and they accepted me as I was.

Work was a different story. I tried to be a good manager during the day, and for the most part I succeeded, primarily because I refused to allow arthritis to be a part of my life while I was at the office. I can honestly say that arthritis did not affect my performance during those early months, even years. However, sometimes, when I'd arrive home late at night, I would literally collapse into bed and cry myself to sleep.

Arthritis can be a progressive disease, and for me the situation naturally worsened. Before long I was lying about my condition and making excuses for being late, or for needing help with the most mundane of tasks. One morning, for example, rather than parking

my car in a public garage and walking the usual two blocks to my office, I called my secretary and asked her to meet me outside the
front door of the office at seven-fifteen so that she could park my
car. So she wouldn't think I was being a complete prima donna, I
told her I had hurt my knee while Rollerblading. She was a wonderful woman and happily obliged. This was the routine for a while, me
faking sports-related injuries and my secretary parking my car.
Eventually, the strain of lying wore on me and I told her the truth.
Her reaction?

"Arthritis? Are you sure? I mean isn't that for *old people?*"

If I had a dollar for every time I heard that—*"Arthritis, isn't that
for old people?"*—I would be a very rich woman today. No such luck,
though. Instead, in those days, I usually just nodded, smiled, mum-
bled some halfhearted response, and went about the business of
being a silent victim. What happens in that situation (and I have
since discovered that it's true of many people with arthritis) is that
you withdraw. You reach a point where you don't even want to tell
people, because you know exactly how they're going to respond. It
just doesn't seem worth the trouble. Better to suffer alone.

I didn't want people at my workplace to pity me or judge me
based on my medical condition. Because I didn't know how to reveal just enough to get the kind of help I needed, without being la-
beled as "the one with arthritis," I chose to be silent. In hindsight,
I realize should have explained to my boss and peers how arthritis
affected me. I should have been specific about what I could and
could not do, and then described the kinds of conditions under
which I would need help. But I didn't, and the weight of the burden
was overwhelming.

My life was a fantasy, and yet a charade. By day I was a corporate
climber, acting as though I had everything under control, doing all
those things that a young executive is supposed to do. By night I
was a young woman increasingly incapacitated by rheumatoid
arthritis. My knees were the biggest problem. Swollen with fluid,

they felt as if they weighed a thousand pounds a piece; I had a terrible time just swinging them over the edge of the bed at night. I reverted to sleeping in the fetal position because there was less discomfort when my joints were bent. Much later I learned that this is one of the worst things you can do if you're suffering from arthritis. When you don't stretch the muscles, the joint can become locked in a specific position, resulting in muscle atrophy and further joint deterioration. So, ironically, even though there is short-term relief—you're able to sleep through the night or get through an afternoon at your desk—long-term damage is being done to the body. Today I'm very cognizant of how I sit, stand, walk ... even sleep. I make a conscious effort to do range-of-motion exercises and straighten my joints as often as possible.

Back then I never gave it a thought. One evening I arrived at my apartment complex, after a long day of work, and was horrified to realize that I couldn't even get out of my car. Exhausted, in excruciating pain, I sat behind the wheel in the parking lot and sobbed. An hour passed before another car pulled in alongside me. I heard a knock at the window and looked up to see Ron's face. He mouthed the words "What's wrong?"

I rolled down the window. "Ron," I cried. "I can't get out of the car."

That was all he needed to hear. Ron opened the door, lifted me out of the car, and carried me upstairs into my apartment. On that night, as Ron pulled back the covers and placed me carefully, gently in bed, I came to the realization that arthritis was beginning to take over my life, and that I had better find a way to fight back.

Dr. Louis Kramer, chief of medical staff at Cedars-Sinai Medical Center in Los Angeles, was my rheumatologist and like a father to me. Our respect for each other went beyond the typical doctor-patient relationship. I trusted him with my life. He was like family. One of the things Dr. Kramer suggested was an experimental procedure known as plasmapheresis.

"None of the traditional medications seem to be working," he said, stating the obvious. "So let's give it a try."

"What's involved?" I asked.

"We'll put you in the hospital for a couple of days at a time, filter out different parts of your blood, and then put it back in your body." He paused. "I have to be honest; it's highly experimental. Your insurance should pay for part of it, though, and if not, we'll work some kind of a deal."

This was my introduction to the world of experimental medicine and clinical trials; it was my first experience as a guinea pig. To be perfectly honest, I was not terribly well-informed about the whole process, and I've since discovered that being informed is of paramount importance. But I also remember thinking, *No matter how crazy it sounds to me, I want to try this, because I'm desperate.* Although today there are credible websites (like the U.S. National Institutes of Health's www.ClinicalTrials.gov) that provide information about clinical trials, it is generally up to your physician to inform you about appropriate clinical trials for which you qualify.

Still, I asked what I thought were the right questions.

"Is it likely to work?"

The doctor shrugged. "I don't know. All I can tell you is, we have nothing to lose. You're young and you want to return to an active lifestyle, right?"

"Uh-huh."

"Well, then, this is what I suggest. But it has to be your decision."

He was right, of course. The ball was in my court. It would take years to develop an ear for these types of conversations, and to understand the ramifications of decisions large and small. Now, when I ask about the side effects of a particular course of treatment, and the response is "Not much, and don't worry because you'll be monitored in the hospital, anyway," I know enough to be skeptical. The truth is, with any experimental treatment, you never know what may happen. To say that you should do your homework before taking part in a clinical trial is to state the obvious. But that's not enough. You also have to be aware of your own psychological and emotional condition; you have to know your own medical history and be prepared to detect the changes that can occur in your body. When the doctor recommends a clinical trial (or any other radical or experimental procedure) because, in his opinion, your choices are "this or nothing," do you believe him? Is it true for you? Because if it is, that pretty much puts all your eggs in the "this" basket, as opposed to the "nothing" basket. "Nothing" is the status quo, and for me, at that time, the status quo was unacceptable.

You have to be aware of who you are and where you stand on the long road to recovery. You have to weigh the risks and the benefits. When the doctor says, "Don't worry about the side effects, they're minimal," stop him. Today, before any trial, I'll bluntly say, "Tell me exactly what the side effects are, and then give me something to read on the subject so that I can take it home and explore it further."

Admittedly, it's hard to make a clear, informed decision when you're in such terrible pain. The power to say yes, to do something proactive about your illness, is right there in front of you. You can run away from the pain and toward hope. That's what clinical trials are all about: hope. From the point of view of the scientist or physician, clinical trials are about research, but from the patient's point of view they represent something much more important: a chance for a healthy life. The physician is in a powerful position in this relationship, because the patient, in many cases, will do anything to alleviate the pain. There have been times during my struggle with arthritis when if someone had said, "We'll cut off your foot to stop the pain in your arm," I might well have responded with "Slice away!" As an advisor to the National Institute of Arthritis and Musculoskeletal and Skin Diseases (NIAMS), I now have a better understanding of the whole paradigm. We need volunteers to take part in clinical trials, no question about it, but we also need physicians who are more sensitive to the vulnerability of their patients. Ultimately, though, the responsibility rests with the individual. As a patient you have to make sure you are aware of all options and risks; not only that, you must understand your own expectations and what motivates you to say yes or no.

For me, the answer was yes. After consulting with my family, but without telling any of my friends or co-workers, I checked into Cedars-Sinai Hospital and hoped for the best. The plan called for twenty-two sessions of blood filtering over the course of approximately one month. They would do one session a day for two consecutive days, give my veins a day off to recover, and then begin the procedure all over again. At the end of the treatment, theoretically, plasma or fluid from my blood would be removed mechanically and replaced with other fluids, and I would be left with several quarts of pure, high-octane, arthritis-free blood.

Alas, things did not go exactly as planned.

I was taken into a room typically used for dialysis (since much of the equipment used in my treatment was the same). There, tubelike needles—I referred to them as "straws" because they were so thick—were inserted into my arms. The blood was drawn out of one arm, circulated through a machine, and the remainder pumped back into the other arm. In a normal patient, the process of plasmapheresis takes about one hour. But I was not a normal person. Small by any reasonable standard, I had in recent months found food increasingly unappealing, and thus become the Incredible Shrinking Woman. By the time I entered the hospital to have my blood filtered, I weighed less than ninety pounds, which meant I had to be fitted with a device known as a pediatric filtering cup. This slowed the filtering process dramatically, so much so that a single session of plasmapheresis consumed more than four hours! By the end of the first session, I was delirious—not just tired, but almost amnesiac. I was in a complete fog.

I spent that night in the hospital. The next morning, when they wheeled me into the dialysis room for a second session, I was reasonably calm and confident, even as they were inserting the needles into my arms. *Been there, done that. No big deal.* Within a few minutes, though, a cold sensation crept over my entire body. I started to shake and shiver. My head began to spin and my vision blurred. The next thing I knew, people were scurrying around the room, shouting and barking out instructions.

"Call the doctor!" I heard one of the nurses say. Apparently, he had already left the room. I felt a needle prick on my thigh, this one smaller, and then everything went black.

When I woke, several hours later, I was back in my room, surrounded by doctors and nurses. What had happened, they explained, was that I had experienced a reaction of some sort, and my body had gone into shock. Just a temporary thing, mind you, and nothing to worry about. It was all under control now. Just to be on the safe side, though, they would be keeping me in the hospital for a few days, at least until the next session was complete.

With the help of an answering service, I was able to get through the entire ordeal without missing too much work, and without revealing my secret to the entire world. I'd wake up at seven in the morning, go to the hospital, have my blood sucked out through a milk-shake straw, go into work for a few hours, then do it again the next day.

At the end of month, to my great disappointment, I felt basically the same, except that my arms, which were covered with track marks (I looked like a junkie!), hurt like crazy. Undaunted, the doctors suggested I try another, similar process called lymphoplasmapheresis. Same idea, they said, only this time they'd be filtering out lymphocyte cells.

"Why not?" I said. "Nothing to lose."

By the end of the first twenty-two-session course of lympho-plasmapheresis, I detected subtle improvement, so we decided to go ahead with a second round. Another month and twenty-two more sessions later, I was a new woman. More precisely, I was an old woman, the old Amye Leong, the one who liked to swim and run and climb trees and play tennis and golf. I'm not exaggerating—the improvement was that significant. It was as if the inflammation had been squeezed out of my body. I couldn't believe it! I had a new lease on life!

One of the first things I did was call my friend Carol and suggest we play some tennis. But it wasn't enough to merely pull a racket out of storage and meet at a local park. No, we had to take a weekend trip to La Costa, a gorgeous golf and tennis resort near San Diego. This was silly, of course, but how can I explain it except to say that I felt as if some part of me had been reborn. A lot of what most people experience with arthritis is about loss, and I was no different. With arthritis, you rarely mourn what you lose. You don't say, "Oh, I miss playing golf . . . I miss playing tennis . . . good-bye swimming." You just stop doing those things one day. You feel bad, naturally, but you don't really mourn, in part because there's too much pain and variation. One day you may be able to do what you like, the next day you may not. When I felt suddenly better, I wanted everything back. And I wanted it right away!

This entire experience was like something out of a science fiction movie—the torturous treatment, the rejuvenation, and, finally, inevitably, the return of symptoms. Our first day in San Diego was wonderful. On the second day I noticed some changes. The aches were returning. I was getting tired. On the tennis court, without warning, I dropped the racket.

"Maybe this is too strenuous," Carol suggested. "Let's try golf." Before long, golf clubs were sailing down the fairways at beautiful

La Costa Country Club, so flimsy and weak was my grip. *This is not good*, I thought. *This is not good at all. C'mon, Amye, get a grip!*

That night I woke from a sound sleep, my body practically on fire. I was having trouble breathing. My knees were throbbing. My hands ached. It was like having the worst case of the flu imaginable.

I called out to Carol, who was sharing a room with me. "Something is not right," I said. "I'm scared."

"What do you mean?"

"I mean I'm falling apart. I don't feel well. I think I need to get to a hospital."

As I dressed, and later, in the car, on the way to Cedars-Sinai, I could almost feel my body aging. It was as though I was going through my battle with arthritis all over again, and this time it wasn't happening over the course of several years—it was happening, literally, in minutes. Never in my life had I been so frightened.

I spent two and a half weeks at Cedars-Sinai, recovering from what they described as a "massive flare." They pumped me up with large doses of prednisone, but there would be no more plasmapheresis or lymphoplasmapheresis. As it turned out, I had experienced something known as "antibody rebound." I had gone through all these sessions of blood filtering, but as fast as the doctors and technicians were removing the bad stuff, my body was manufacturing new stuff. The disease, in other words, was coming back, and stronger than ever.

Some months later one of my rheumatology friends suggested I attend a conference at UCLA Medical Center, where someone was presenting a paper on experimental medical treatments. I arrived late and took a seat in the back row. The doctor at the podium was talking about plasmapheresis and lymphoplasmapheresis, and he was discussing a case in which a young woman had experienced a particularly gruesome episode of antibody rebound. When a patient goes through plasmapheresis, the doctor explained, she must be placed on some type of nonsteroidal anti-inflammatory drug. If not, the patient would experience marked improvement for a short period of time, and then all symptoms would suddenly return. This, he said, was antibody rebound. And, of course, he was talking about me. I had been a test case, one for the books.

Despite this one very bad experience, I was not through with experimental treatments. Far from it. In fact, in the months following my horrifying introduction to antibody rebound, I embraced all manner of alternative therapies: acupuncture; vitamin B_{12} injections; herbal therapy. A distant relative in Hong Kong was kind enough, or disturbed enough, to send me marijuana soaked in alcohol—I wasn't sure whether to smoke it or drink it. (It was actually supposed be placed on the affected joint to draw out the inflammation.) That I actually refused to do, because it just seemed ridiculous, and vaguely immoral, if not downright illegal. I tried DMSO (dimethylsulfoxide, a medication applied topically that the medical community hailed as a pain relief miracle), which did nothing except remove the top two layers of my skin. I tried holistic medicine, in which the ends of my hair were cut off and evaluated to determine my body chemistry. I gobbled handfuls of little white pills—dietary supplements—as part of a homeopathic program. I attended séances. I visited fortune-tellers. I tried everything . . . even faith healing.

I had heard of a Baptist revival at the Pasadena Civic Auditorium. While I told my family I was going to see a faith healer, I didn't tell my friends because I could only imagine the reaction it would have provoked. Still, I was willing to give it a try. In fact, I was willing to throw myself into it. That's something I've learned over the years— if you're going to try new or experimental therapies or any therapy, do it with gusto. If you don't believe in the treatment, if you *can't* believe in it, then don't bother. Science is only now showing us that the power of our beliefs actually makes a difference. That's true of the biologics, the COX-2s, the immunosuppressive drugs, or even marijuana soaked in alcohol. You must believe there is a chance for success before you embark on a course of treatment. The attitude is important, the belief system matters; that's been proven time and time again in studies, and it's one of the reasons patients often experience an alleviation of symptoms when taking nothing more than a placebo. The mind, after all, has remarkable recuperative power.

So I headed off to the revival. I got in the car, said a little prayer, and started driving. I didn't even have directions, hadn't ever been to Pasadena, and so had only a vague notion of where I was headed. Somehow, though, I found the Pasadena Civic Auditorium, a bit of luck that I hoped represented some sort of omen. When I walked inside, the auditorium was packed, maybe three or four thousand people. The preacher was on stage, standing in front of a long line of people, all of them swaying and humming, as if lost in some transcendental state. I watched incredulously as the preacher walked down the line, whispered something to each person and placed a hand on each forehead. Then, one by one, each person crumbled to the floor of the stage, as if unconscious. People were dropping like flies, falling all over the place. Although I wanted to believe, I couldn't help but smirk.

Right! What a bunch of fakers.

And yet, I went up anyway. It's hard to explain, but about two and a half hours into this three-hour revival, there I was, at the end of a long line snaking its way toward the preacher. As the line grew shorter, my skepticism weakened; more than that, I actually became part of the flock. If this didn't work, it wasn't going to be because of my doubt. "I believe . . . ," I whispered under my breath. "I believe."

One by one the parishioners fell, until there were only a few people between the faith healer and me. I could see him coming closer, see him sweating, working, preaching.

"I believe . . . I believe . . . I believe . . ."

Once in a while the image of my friends intruded. I imagined them sitting in the front row, shaking their heads. But I pushed them aside and pressed on.

"I believe . . . I believe . . . I believe . . ."

Suddenly the preacher was in front of me, asking me what was wrong. His hair was matted, his face flushed red, his suit drenched with perspiration.

"I have rheumatoid arthritis," I said numbly.

He nodded, touched me on the forehead, and began to talk loudly, with his eyes closed. "God is going to save you! God will make you better! *You are healed!"*

He pushed me hard, drove me right to the ground, or at least into the arms of one of his assistants, whose job clearly was to make sure that I found the floor safely and quickly. I closed my eyes and remained prone for a few minutes, until someone tapped me on the shoulder and helped me to my feet. As I walked back to my seat, I felt tingly, although I now attribute that to the fact that I was on stage, in front of a few thousand people, which alone is a bit of a rush. Everyone was so jubilant. I didn't want to be the one to spoil the party. But I did notice right away that my knees still ached, and my hands were sore. There was no discernible difference in my condition.

Okay, don't give up. Maybe it'll kick in on the way home.

But it didn't. Nothing happened, nothing changed. In fact, within a couple of months I would be alone in a soiled bed in my apartment in Marina del Rey, waiting for a ride to the hospital. But the lesson I learned was this: My own attitude is of immeasurable importance. The denial I'd been experiencing was just Amye fighting Amye. If I was going to get a grip on this disease, I needed to be enthusiastically involved—whether in prayer or belief or medication. Whatever the next step, I had to be focused on a positive effort to get better. I had to be aware of my own foibles, willing to listen to all options, and take the primary responsibility for change.

7

Alone No More

This old guy wobbles into an ice cream shop. He has a hard time walking. He's hunched over, shuffling slowly, a pained expression on his face. The old man goes up to the counter and says, in a thin, weak voice, "Banana split, please."

The lady at the counter looks at him, smiles compassionately, and says, "Crushed nuts?"

The old man shakes his head.

"No . . . Arthritis!"

On the night of my Marina del Rey meltdown, the night when I ruined a perfectly good set of sheets, I wound up in the emergency room of Daniel Freeman Hospital in Inglewood, California. For the better part of forty-eight hours I was confined to a bed with intravenous lines pumping fluids and electrolytes back into my body, while the medical staff tried to figure out what to do with me. I wanted to go home, of course, though I really didn't have the energy to dispute anyone's advice or recommendation. On the second day, I was told there was no way that the hospital could discharge me back to my apartment, because to do so would be grossly irresponsible.

"Then what do we do?" I asked.

"You're in bad shape," one of the doctors said. "You need to be admitted to our arthritis rehabilitation program."

At first I said, "No!" but my will quickly subsided. "What exactly is it?" I asked.

"It's a three-week hospital program that will help you get your body back in shape and get your arthritis under control. But it's going to take time. It's not just an acute-care kind of thing. You'll need patience, dedication, strength."

Great. I'm oh-for-three.

"How long would I have to be here?" I asked.

The doctor shrugged, turned his palms up as if to say, "I don't know," though clearly he had an idea. "Three weeks at least," he said. "Maybe longer."

My mind fairly reeled with all the reasons why I couldn't possibly spend the better part of the next month in a hospital. There were bills to pay, withering friendships that were in serious need of nurturing. I was very concerned about my job, my career, because I had already missed so much time in the preceding months while going through plasmapheresis. I was worried about my own ability to make a physical and emotional commitment to this program of therapy. In the end, though, I lacked the resolve to decline the invitation. I was exhausted, scared, and sick.

"Okay," I agreed. "I'll do it."

They gave me thirty-six hours to get my affairs in order. I was discharged from the emergency room and, with the help of my parents and my sister, returned to my apartment and prepared for life as a hospital patient. Mom and Dad hadn't seen me in a few months, and when they arrived from Bakersfield that afternoon they were appropriately stunned by my appearance. My weight upon discharge from the emergency room was a scant seventy-nine pounds. There were track marks all over my arms from the IV needles and the plasmapheresis. My hair was unruly, my skin a ghostly pallor. They had known I was ill, but they didn't know the extent of my illness. Here was their daughter, once so vivacious and driven and energetic, slumped in a wheelchair, her hands and feet gnarled, her body a bag of bones.

There wasn't a lot of talking or soul baring in those thirty-six hours, mainly because there was too much work to be done. Like models of efficiency, everyone went about the task of getting Amye on the road to recovery. The plan was to put all my belongings in storage, sublet my beautiful swinging-singles apartment, and check me into the rehabilitation unit at Daniel Freeman Hospital . . . for as long as necessary. I sat in a wheelchair, barely able to keep my eyes open, as my parents and sister packed everything up. Mom and Dad took all my personal items and drove them back up to Bakersfield; my sister took my car and refrigerator. J then drove me to the hospital, helped me register and get settled in my room, and then gave me a big hug and a kiss and said good-bye.

As J walked out, I slumped on the hospital bed, too weak to sit up, and thought about where I was and how I had come to be there, and how long this might be my new home. The rehab section was less drab than a normal hospital, with bright yellow walls and floral curtains. Still, there was no mistaking that it was a hospital. The antiseptic smell, the constant clattering of trays and chairs and equipment, the incessant drone of voices—all made the setting instantly recognizable as a place where people came because they could no longer take of themselves.

The first few days were really all about fear, about being babied and coddled and convinced that I belonged precisely where I was. Arthritis, in effect, was shoved down my throat. After all the years of hiding the disease, of avoiding rather than fighting it, I was now compelled to acknowledge its hold on me. I was forced to admit that I hadn't taken care of myself, and that my own stubbornness was at least partially responsible for my current state of health. My first roommate was an elderly woman (come to think of it, all of my hospital roommates were elderly women), and yet, for most of the first week I spent more time in bed than she did. I would watch sadly as she was dressed and escorted to various other areas. I was so weak that I could barely move. I remember on one of the first mornings trying to sit up in bed . . . and falling over sideways because I didn't have the strength to prop up the pillows correctly. A nurse walked into the room, took one look at me, tipping pathetically toward the edge of the bed, and said, with a pitiful smile, "Oh, honey, you are really in bad shape, aren't you?"

As I nodded feebly, my eyes welled with tears. I was overcome with emotion, for this was the first time that someone I didn't even know had looked at me objectively and immediately identified the depth of my illness. She smacked me right in the face with the reality of my condition.

You are really in bad shape.

It hit me then, perhaps for the first time: I was a victim. I was so sad and in so much pain, because this disease, rheumatoid arthritis, had been consuming me—physically and emotionally. Even though I had done little things, like reaching out to my parents, and to my friend Tina, this was the very first time that someone else had recognized the severity of my condition and mirrored for me just how bad it really was. I could see it in her eyes, and that image made me lose control of my emotions. I burst into tears and began sobbing uncontrollably. The nurse walked over to my bed and wrapped her arms around me.

"That's all right," she said. "We're going to make you better."

She was making a promise, and while I didn't doubt her sincerity, I was nonetheless saddened by the fact that I needed her help, and the help of so many other people. Arthritis had made me a victim, and I *hated* being a victim. Being a victim means having something done to you that you have no control over. You're powerless. It's like being attacked from behind—you have no opportunity to defend yourself, to put up your arms and fight back. That's what arthritis did to me: it assaulted me, hurt me, crippled me.

Today I do not consider myself a victim of arthritis. I was able to stand up to this disease. That doesn't mean I don't experience pain anymore. There are still days when I can't move very well. But I have decided to take back control of my life. I make decisions about my treatment. I've become an advocate for myself and for others who live with arthritis. And when I'm faced with a challenge, I meet it head-on and fight to overcome it.

I was able to move beyond being a victim by tapping into a reserve of strength I didn't know I had. You can do this, too. Look within yourself and realize that you are a person of worth and have the capacity to be of value to others. Determine what you want to achieve and believe that you deserve it. Finally, know without a doubt, that you are stronger than the arthritis. I'm not saying this will be easy to do. It took me years to discover this for myself. But I urge you to call on your stores of faith and perseverance to discover your internal strength, so that you too will no longer be victimized by arthritis.

If the first couple of weeks of my stay at Daniel Freeman were about getting Amye back on her feet (so to speak—in reality I was still confined to a wheelchair), the third week was about honest-to-goodness rehabilitation. It was then that an army of people began filing through my room on a daily basis, saying things like, "Hi, I'm Muriel, your occupational therapist." Or, "Hi, I'm Roberta, your nurse-practitioner." My friend Tina was a physical therapist at Daniel Freeman, and she asked to be assigned to my case, which was nice, because at least there was one familiar face each day. But in general I felt like a specimen of some sort, an object to be wheeled from one place to another by smiling strangers. That was my take on it, anyway, and it stemmed as much from a generally surly outlook on life as it did from a realistic interpretation of the situation. When you're confined to a hospital setting, it's easy to get discouraged, grumpy, even hostile. You never know who's going to walk through the door, and you don't have any control over it. Someone barges into your room, stands at the foot of your bed, and begins to have a discussion with you. Or someone wakes you from a sound sleep and says, "Hi, Amye, how are you? And you open a heavy, medicated eyelid and say something like "Lousy . . . that's why I'm here. Who are you?"

Little did I know at the time that each one of these people knew exactly what he or she was doing, that they in fact represented one of the very best rehabilitative staffs in the United States. I had the incredibly good fortune to be a patient at Daniel Freeman in one of the two consecutive years when it was ranked as the number-one rehabilitation program in the country, not only for trauma, but for arthritis as well. To say I was in good hands would be a colossal understatement.

Not that I was grateful. Oh, no. It would be several more weeks before I would reach that stage of enlightenment. For me, the introduction to arthritis therapy was a bumpy, unpleasant, unnerving, intrusive, and dehumanizing experience. It was all necessary and indisputably beneficial but I was, for the most part, a reluctant and cranky patient. For one thing, I found the schedule to be utterly exhausting. At seven each morning the nurses would come in and wake me. By seven-thirty my breakfast was sitting on a tray in front of me. They would help me open containers; sometimes they'd have to literally spoon the food into my mouth because I was so severely flared that my fingers couldn't hold a fork or spoon. At eight I'd get a sponge bath. At eight-thirty a nurse would transfer me to a wheelchair and say, "Okay, we're off to physical therapy."

Even though I had a friend who worked as a physical therapist, I didn't really understand the concept. Not until I became a patient. I'd be wearing two flimsy hospital gowns—one covering the front, one covering the back—as they wheeled me to physical therapy. Once there, I'd be hooked up to a harness and hoisted into the air, not unlike a fallen horse after surgery. Then they'd slowly lower me into a big tub of warm water, where Tina would work with me. Although I found the whole process of preparing for this therapy to be degrading, I soon came to realize its benefits. Unable to walk or even stand for the previous few weeks, I was amazed and delighted to discover that I could stand with relative ease in warm water. Like a fish being returned to the sea, I felt instantly at home. The warmth of the water (about one hundred degrees) soothed my aching joints, and the buoyancy supported my weight. In that setting, Tina and I worked on passive assistance exercises. She would slowly, carefully, gently move my arms and legs through the water. It was painful, no doubt about it; here I was moving and bending joints I hadn't moved in some time, and they naturally resisted her efforts. The idea was to work my muscles, to improve range of motion, to nourish the joints through movement and exercise.

When you have arthritis, it's easy to be so consumed by pain that you give up and resign yourself to a life without movement, but that's just about the worst thing you can do. I learned at Daniel Freeman Hospital that physical therapy is an extremely important weapon in the battle against arthritis. I discovered that in order for joints to be healthy, they need exercise. I'm not talking about running ten miles a day. I'm talking about motion, pure and simple. For so much of the previous month—indeed, for so many *years*—pain had been a moderating factor for me. It told me not to move. It screamed at my joints: *"Stop! You'll be sorry!"* In truth, it is submitting to these messages that will leave you with regret. No matter how much it hurts, you have to keep moving. You have to nourish your joints or they will forget their purpose. They'll shorten and

compress, and they'll become as brittle and fragile as dry rubber
bands.

Occupational therapy initially did not win my approval quite as
easily. I didn't understand the concept, and I was usually so exhausted from a morning of physical therapy that I had little energy
or enthusiasm left over. "OT" began with one-on-one sessions, just
me and a therapist doing a lot of evaluation, trying to determine
how well I could bend my wrists (not well), how high I could lift my
arm (not very high), the level of dexterity in my fingers (extremely
limited). After a few days I was moved, like all patients, into a group
environment. My introduction to this setting went badly, thanks to
my poor attitude. I was wheeled into a huge, open area with a lot of
tables, counter space, and what appeared to be a bunch of toys.
The occupational therapist's job was to help me develop a sense of
pride and accomplishment through the completion of various tasks,
most of which were supposed to be enjoyable. At the same time, by
learning to master these tasks, I'd be improving my range of motion
and giving my beleaguered joints a workout. It was all clearly explained to me, and it made sense. Nevertheless, I wanted no part of
it. My attitude wasn't just bad; it was bilious. When I looked around
this room and saw what appeared to be a senior citizens' center,
with a dozen or so white-haired women sitting in their wheelchairs,
hunched over tables, doing some kind of handicraft, I wanted to
bolt straight for the door.

Needless to say, I wasn't capable of *bolting* anywhere. I found myself at a table with a group of these women, seated at a spot that had
clearly been reserved for me. A glance around the room told me I
was at least three decades younger than anyone else there, with
the exception of the occupational therapist, who said to me, in that
annoyingly cheery tone that everyone in this place seemed to have
mastered, "Well, Amye, what would *you* like to do today?"

"I don't want to do anything," I sneered.

Unfazed, the OT said, "That's fine. You can just watch."

Meanwhile, all these old women were chatting away, trying to have fun, and firing all kinds of questions at me:

"Hi, are you new to the group?"

"How long have you been here?"

"You look too young to have arthritis. How old are you, dear?"

That last one, in particular, fed my bad attitude: *I do not belong here! I'm just passing through, ladies. I'm only here because I happen to have a disease that people like you are supposed to get. So get out of my face!*

Oh, but were they persistent. Nothing could upset them, nothing could fluster them. Certainly they weren't going to be put off by a surly young woman in a wheelchair. They kept talking among themselves, occasionally trying to drag me into the conversation, and they continually fiddled with their various projects and crafts. They were so sweet, and I was unrelentingly sour.

"Grace, isn't Amye pretty? And she's so young."

"I know . . . the poor dear."

I looked at the clock. I'd only been in the room about fifteen minutes. *God help me. What am I doing in this place, and how do I get out?*

I sat there for more than half an hour until I was completely bored out of my wits. Finally, just to stay awake, I turned to a woman named Helen, who was working with some tiles, and said, sort of sharply, "What are you doing there?"

Helen smiled. "I'm making a mosaic. Would you like to try it?"

I shrugged. "All right."

The occupational therapist came right over and placed some materials in front of me. In retrospect, I can see now that she knew precisely what she was doing, as did everyone on that staff. Many occupational therapists have a keen knowledge of psychology and motivation, because it's not at all unusual to encounter patients with the same sort of resistive attitude I displayed. Let's put it bluntly: I was not nice in that session, but the OT was right there for me when I started to come around. She brought me some ceramic tiles, and I tried at once to pick up the tiny tiles. But I found out that what Helen was doing so effortlessly was not so easy for me. I needed Helen's help to lift the tiles onto my work space. I needed all of their help to understand what I was experiencing.

Over the next few weeks, as I let my guard down around these women, I came to understand that I was sicker than any of them. Interestingly, though, in that room it wasn't about illness; it was about a process of socialization that involved redirecting anger and hostility, and maybe teaching the mind how to think differently so that you could create something on your own. It was a creative problem-solving process within a supportive group setting, and I was amazed to see how well it worked.

I started out by making a little trivet about four inches square. The other women taught me how to put pieces of tile together to form a colorful pattern. I caulked it, dried it, painted it. Within a week I had created something beautiful, and I felt so proud. Through occupational therapy, and with the help of these other women, I began to experience a shift within myself, a move toward an understanding. I realized that arthritis had torn me down completely, emotionally and spiritually. My response was to lash out at the world. Now I understood that I had to be gracious first to myself—to give myself credit for some small sense of accomplishment. That small trivet, created and completed by Amye Leong, was my first significant accomplishment in spite of arthritis. It represented a coalescing of my fears, laying them on the trivet, examining them, and acknowledging that it was okay to be afraid. This experience was about *me*. I had to start asking questions. I had to reach out to other people. It was true that arthritis had been foisted upon me, that it had victimized me, but now I had an opportunity, even an obligation, to take control of my own care. That process started there, at Daniel Freeman Hospital in Inglewood, California.

Never before had I really talked with anyone about my arthritis in great depth; at least, not with anyone who understood. There is something to be said for support groups, for sharing experiences and feelings and stories, for sharing laughter and tears, with people who understand in a fundamental way what your journey has been like. All these women were older than my mother, and yet the generation gap was bridged by our commonality, by our shared experience of arthritis.

Today, there is much research to support the value and benefits of self-help, mutual aid, or support groups. To communicate honestly, without bias or fear of retribution, with others who share a similar challenge carries with it a sense of mastery over the challenge, reducing stress, improving practical education, and even reducing in-hospital care.

Reluctant to the point of obstinance in the beginning, I later came to embrace and enjoy my group counseling sessions with these gentle ladies. We would gather with a psychologist and talk about what it was that had brought us to this place and this point in time. We talked about goals and what it would be like when we returned to the outside world. I learned how to measure pain in these sessions, how to grade it on a scale of one to ten. I learned about assistive devices, tools that I could use to comb my hair and brush my teeth. Every woman (and every man, I'm sure) feels an obligation to make herself presentable, to do her duty in the bathroom each day: take a shower, comb her hair, brush her teeth, fix her makeup, etc. The ability to complete this routine had slipped from my grasp, and I had let my personal appearance deteriorate. I didn't always brush my teeth, and I didn't always comb my hair. I had always taken such pride in looking presentable, and now I had lost that, too. So to be presented with devices that made it possible to correct that situation, to have control over my hygiene and appearance . . . that was heartening.

The assistive devices were introduced on the twentieth day of my stay. By then it had become clear that I would not be getting discharged after the usual three-week course of treatment; I was in for a long haul. The rehabilitation and treatment intensified with each passing day. There were weekly meetings with my entire medical team: a rheumatologist, physical therapist, occupational therapist, psychologist, and nurse. They would talk about me as if I were the center of their world. They talked in terms that I could understand, using clinical terms and then explaining them to me. Always, in the end, I would be drawn into the conversation and my input would be solicited. I came to understand that I was an important part—maybe the most important part—of my own health-care team, because they based many of their decisions on the information they received from me. This had a profound effect on me, because it was the start of a management system, one with multiple parts. Previously, there had been only chaos in my arthritis treatment; now I could see order, logic, progress.

Today, the concept of an in-hospital multidisciplinary arthritis team is virtually defunct, thanks mainly to managed health care, but I think having a group of specialists—each with his or her own perspective—working together to manage your arthritis treatment is vital. Ideally, you should have: a rheumatologist to manage your medical treatment; a physical therapist to evaluate your strength and function and determine what exercises will keep you strong, flexible, and active; an occupational therapist to help you master the activities of daily living; a dietician or nutritionist who understands how foods interact with medications and what foods are beneficial for you; and a psychologist, counselor, support group, or even a good friend, to help you deal with the anger, fear, frustration, and depression that often accompany a chronic illness. Most important, you have to be the team captain, pulling together all the members of your team and making sure they all work together and remain focused on your care. An invaluable resource is the Arthritis Foundation's Arthritis Self-Help Course (ASHC). This education program teaches you how to become an active partner in your arthritis care. For information about ASHC, call your local chapter of the Arthritis Foundation or visit their website at www.arthritis.org.

My stay at Daniel Freeman stretched out over ninety-three days, and in that time I experienced a lot of ups and downs. The elderly women I initially rejected became my friends, and through those friendships I learned a lot about myself. I shared laughter with a steady stream of roommates, including several nuns (Daniel Freeman is a Catholic hospital). This was an eye-opener, to say the least, especially because I'm not Catholic. Nuns were not the strange and mysterious people I imagined, but rather some of the warmest and funniest people I have ever known. The people most likely to visit a nun in the hospital, of course, are other nuns, and my room often looked like a convent. But it sure didn't sound like a convent, at least not like any convent I'd ever envisioned. You see, I discovered that nuns have a vast repertoire of raunchy jokes, and when in the company of other nuns, they don't hesitate to share these jokes. I was amazed and appalled and entertained all at once. These women were wearing habits and everything, and yet they were telling dirty jokes! I couldn't believe it! On more than one occasion they made me laugh so hard that I nearly cried. And they would always leave me with a hug and a prayer and a wish for good health. Strange thing, too: my joints always felt a little bit better after they left. I think that was when I first realized the value of humor in fighting illness.

By about seven weeks, although I was still in bad shape physically, I was in a better place attitudinally. I was buying into the educational process, in part because I had begun to forge friendships with the people who were helping me. They weren't just therapists anymore; they were people who cared about me, and about whom I cared. I liked my older roommates and partners in group therapy, but I longed to spend time with people closer to my own age, so I began to socialize not only with Tina but also with many of the other health-care personnel. I'd ask them to stop by my room for lunch, just to talk. Tina told me there were other young patients in another part of the rehabilitation unit, in the trauma center, and one afternoon she wheeled me down and just left me there, surrounded by patients, all quite young, who had experienced horrific injuries: broken bones, spinal injuries, head trauma. Most had been involved in automobile accidents. One minute they were fine; the next minute they were here, encased in plaster or hooked up to machines that made it possible for them to breathe or go to the bathroom. I can't tell you how much it helped me to meet some of these young people. We talked about trauma and the shock of being young and suddenly losing what had once seemed to be a fundamental part of our existence. We talked about feeling cheated and angry and marginalized. My experiences with those other young patients would eventually serve as the impetus for a decision to establish a support group for young people with arthritis. At the time, though, it served a much more practical purpose: it gave me companionship, a sense of perspective. It helped me heal.

I learned that it didn't matter how we had gotten here. We were all young, our bodies didn't work as they were supposed to, and we were in physical and emotional pain. We shared a camaraderie and took comfort in the fact that we were not alone on this journey. We cheered each other's minuscule accomplishments and were elated to share the next milestone of our recovery and rehabilitation.

Undeniably, though, there were bad days, like the time Muriel came to get me for occupational therapy and I was in a foul mood.

"We're going to do something different today," she said.

"Uh-uh," I grumbled. "I don't feel like it. I'm tired."

Muriel laughed. "Sorry, kid." She began wheeling me through the hospital corridors, faster than usual, as if she was excited about something. Finally we reached the end of a long corridor, and with a tremendous *whump!* (just the way it sounds when they're frantically wheeling a gurney around the bloody halls of *ER*) she pushed me right through the double doors into the occupational therapy suite. When I looked up I saw a group of men in penguin suits—tuxedos—and some other people with cameras, and one tall, thin guy dressed in leather from head to toe. He had thick, dark hair and big, piercing eyes, and he walked right up to me.

"Hi, my name is David. I understand your name is Amye."

"Yeah . . . whatever." I was feeling tired and sick and I was angry with Muriel for forcing me to do something I didn't want to do, so I was in no mood to play along. Besides, I had no idea who this guy was. He certainly was persistent, though.

"Amye," he said, "how would you like to learn a magic trick?"

"Why?"

He looked around the room, smiled, and looked back at me. Obviously he was accustomed to dealing with tough audiences. "Because it might be kind of fun."

"All right . . . go ahead," I said with a sigh.

He took out a piece of rope, and with long, magnificent fingers, like the fingers of a musician, he proceeded to cut it into several pieces. His hands worked swiftly, smoothly, efficiently. It was mesmerizing. Well, you probably know the trick—the magician somehow puts the pieces of rope back together and creates a long single strand, free of knots, right there in full view of the audience. And that's what this guy did.

"How did you do that?" I asked. I have to admit, even though it's an old trick, he did it so flawlessly that you couldn't help but be impressed.

The magician gave me a little wink. "Pretty cool, huh? Want to learn how to do it?"

"Uhhhh . . . sure."

And just like that, David Copperfield had made a new fan. At the time I didn't know he was the international entertainer and magician and, to be honest, I'm not sure I would have recognized the name even if someone had told me. Although he was already a big hit in Las Vegas and just starting to host his annual television specials, he was not the worldwide celebrity he is today.

It turned out that David was launching something called Project Magic, a rehabilitation program for hospitals with a partnership between professional magicians and occupational therapists. The concept was brilliant: as part of an overall rehabilitation program, magic would be used to build confidence and improve muscle strength and coordination. As you learned a trick, you would get stronger and more confident. It was about practice and movement, repetition and discipline. Certain tricks depended heavily on certain movements and thus exercised specific joints. Theoretically, there would be a trick for every patient, regardless of his or her disability. The program met the twin goals of improving self-esteem and physical rehabilitation. When David came back two weeks later and I demonstrated to him the very same rope trick that he had performed that first day, I swelled with pride. And I loved demonstrating the trick to other people. There's something oddly invigorating about being in a wheelchair and doing a magic trick that your able-bodied audience can't do.

In time David and I became close friends. He took Project Magic to a national level and asked me to be on his board of directors. I also chaired Project Magic's first fund-raiser at the Magic Castle, a fabulous private club for magicians in the Hollywood Hills. I can't say enough about David and his work with Project Magic. Today I am a true believer in the value of occupational therapy and the importance of instilling fun in the learning process.

As my attitude improved, so too did my appetite. My girlfriends would sneak in sushi and other goodies to my hospital room. My parents even took me out on a day pass for some "real" food one afternoon. They assumed I wanted Chinese food, but

I instructed my father to drive straight to Junior's, a nearby Jewish delicatessen for some bagels, lox, and matzo-ball soup!

During my last week in the hospital, representatives from a manufacturer of orthopedic shoes stopped by for a visit. Their task was to fit my deformed feet with walking shoes. The salesman brought in what appeared to be samples of the company's entire catalogue for me to sample. Most of them looked like old granny shoes, with big, chunky souls and thick uppers. They were so hideous that I simply refused to try them on. These were four-hundred-dollar shoes! I couldn't imagine paying that much money for something that ugly. I felt bad enough about my appearance—there was no way I was going to compound matters by wearing ugly old-lady shoes.

"Sorry," I told the salesman near the end of his second day working with me. "I'm not wearing those things, and I'm not buying them!" The poor guy shuffled away, looking like a beaten man. I took no pleasure in making his life difficult, but I did feel as though I had won another tiny battle. I preferred no shoes to those shoes.

It became apparent, as I began to eat more, talk more, laugh more, that discharge was imminent. I had been measuring the passage of time by looking at a jacaranda tree outside my window. The jacaranda is a beautiful purple flowering tree that blossoms gloriously in March, and by June has dropped all its flowers. I had checked into the hospital in March, just as the jacaranda was opening up. I saw this tree flower and bloom, and now, as May gave way to June, the petals were falling. For me this was a real sense of the passing of time; it was at once a sense of loss and accomplishment. I'd lost three months—*ninety-three days!*—of my life to this place, but I'd gained something too. I had grown immeasurably. Now it was time to move on.

I had no idea what the future held. The program at Daniel Freeman was designed to give the patient stability. Stability for me meant no more terrible flares, and a level of pain that was at least tolerable. But it still meant being confined to a wheelchair. My body had been eaten away by this disease, and now I had to learn to function with what was left. Stability still meant "crippled," and discharge meant trading a hospital environment for some other type of assisted-care living arrangement. Because of the type of family in which I was raised, there was never any doubt about what the next step would be, or upon whose shoulders this burden would fall.

I was going home.

8

Home Again

The morning of my ninety-fourth day at Daniel Freeman Hospital began just as the previous ninety-three had: with a wake-up call, a sponge bath, and breakfast in bed. That's where the normality ended. I knew I was being released that morning. It was a warm June Saturday. My parents were on their way down from Bakersfield to pick me up and my doctor would soon be in to make rounds and fill out the discharge papers. One of the funny things about being in a hospital for such a staggeringly long period of time (today, in the era of strict, tight-fisted managed care, a three-month rehabilitation program would be unthinkable in all but the most dire of circumstances) is that you not only outlast a dozen different roommates, but you also outlast some of the employees and you get to know just about everyone on a first-name basis. Believe me, when the kitchen staff routinely says, "Hi, Amye. How's it going?" you know you've been there too long.

But on the ninety-fourth day, as the light came streaming into my room and I looked at the jacaranda tree outside my window, a different feeling swept over me: a feeling of excitement and fear and sadness all rolled into one. It's so easy to become accustomed to your surroundings. There is an emotional and spiritual level of comfort associated with virtually any routine, even if that routine began as something unpleasant, and would still be viewed as unpleasant by most observers. A lot of people, myself included for a while, considered the long-term rehabilitation unit at a place like Daniel Freeman to be something akin to a prison. That's a bit hyperbolic, I know, because prisons are inherently punitive and brutal whereas the good people at Daniel Freeman were sincerely interested in and committed to improving the quality of their patients' lives. Still, from an emotional standpoint, there are similarities. I could not leave the hospital; while there I was kept on a strict schedule, and I relied on others for my most basic needs. My freedom and privacy had been stripped away. I wasn't able to control how or when I got out of bed. I wasn't free to go outside when I pleased. I never knew who would invade my room. I had no control over people turning the lights on and off, or squawking into the intercom next to my bed. I had no control over my environment, and isn't that really a type of prison?

Somehow, though, I became comfortable, if not content, with that scenario. Daniel Freeman Hospital became my home. I adapted. Maybe that's part of my personality. My parents have always said, "Amye, you were such an easy baby. You were happy with whatever we put in front of you." I don't know, maybe I was born with that ability. Maybe to go with whatever gene there is that made me predisposed to arthritis, I also inherited an adaptability gene. God knows, something helped me get through those three months— three months in an environment that can most charitably be described as "challenging."

Somehow, even when faced with such a restrictive set of circumstances, you learn to cope. The mind is extraordinary that way;

you trick yourself into believing that the routine—any routine—is tolerable, just to maintain a grip on your sanity. There are little things you do so you can feel you have even a bit of control. There are small battles you can wage that have a reasonable chance of being won. For example, one of the things I did at Daniel Freeman was ask someone to create a sign for me that said, PLEASE KNOCK BEFORE ENTERING, and I had it hung on the outside of my hospital room door. It was so simple, but it meant so much. One of the worst things about being in a hospital is that loss of privacy. This small gesture—the construction of a handwritten sign—gave me a measure of pride and dignity at a time when I had little of either.

I've talked with hundreds of people with arthritis about the concept of acceptance. A great many of them—and indeed a great many people with any chronic illness—find this to be a distasteful term. They'll say to me, "I will never *accept* arthritis!" They say it with such anger, such passion. I would take issue with that approach. I think the hostility is misdirected. For me, acceptance of my environment, acceptance of my disease, was about understanding the obstacles I faced; it represented a clear awareness that I was, to put it colloquially, in a real pickle. *Accepting* arthritis did not mean *enjoying* it. It meant finding a level of comfort in my own mind, so that I would have some sense of stability and, eventually, a foundation on which I could begin to erect a new life.

By the time I was discharged from Daniel Freeman, in June of 1983, I had come to accept my role as a young woman with rheumatoid arthritis, but I did not yet understand what that really meant, or where the disease would lead me next (I had yet to consider the possibility that I might lead the disease). That morning, a stream of people—nurses, orderlies, therapists—wandered in and out of my room. When I'd tell them I was being discharged, they'd smile, give me a hug, and say something like "Good for you! But we'll miss you here." And you know what? I was going to miss them, too. I had become so close to these people, and now I was leaving. That was the way it worked for them, of course. Patients came into their lives, accepted their care, and moved on. Rarely, however, did anyone stay for ninety-three days. In fact, I left Daniel Freeman arthritis rehab as the official single-stay record holder (and the mark still stands today). For the staff, the job would go on. There would be new patients, but similar work. For me, life was about to change dramatically, and I felt more than a little anxious about it. Just before I left, I looked around the room one last time. I looked into the tiny closet, which held four items of clothing (all I ever needed). I looked in the bathroom. I looked down the hall. I took a deep breath and held it: *I want to remember what this room looks like. I want to remember what it smells like, sounds like. I want to feel it . . . taste it. Because I am never coming back here again!*

My discharge was based on the fact that I had reached a point of "physical stability," which was, after all, the stated goal of the program. But that hardly meant I had recovered. Stability, in my case, still meant being unable to walk. It meant being unable to eat in a restaurant without having people stare at me. It meant having hands and feet that were horribly deformed.

Along with my discharge papers I was given a set of at-home exercises. We're not talking Jane Fonda or Kathy Smith here, folks. We're talking about movements that most able-bodied people would not even consider exercise, like lying on your bed, pointing your toes to the sky, and holding the position for a count of ten. That was the extent of it. I was still in pretty bad shape. I had been dependent in the hospital, and the truth was, I would be dependent when I left the hospital. My mom and dad would have to help me with the simplest of tasks, like washing my hair, cutting my food, even going to the bathroom. It made me feel like a baby. At the same time, there was a level of comfort in knowing that I was going home, back to the same house, the same room, in which I had been raised. A part of me wanted nothing more than for Mommy and Daddy to hold me, protect me, make me feel well again.

There was never any question in my mind or theirs that my parents would care for me. There was always a strong ethic in our household when it came to matters of family and work, and my unfortunate situation fell under both headings. No one ever talked about it; there was never any discussion of "options." There was an assumption that Amye would need help, and Mom and Dad would be the ones to provide that help.

I can't deny feeling a vast range of conflicting emotions as I lay in the seat of my parents' Volvo on the two-hour ride to Bakersfield. With the windows down, the California air cooling my joints, and the mountains rolling by in the distance, I said to myself, *This feels pretty good.* On the other hand, I was a young adult who was retreating into the past. All my friends were deep into their careers, making good money, getting married, raising families, and here I was going back to the nest, admitting that I was incapable of caring for myself. This was hard stuff.

There are no set rules for dealing with the sudden presence of a caregiver in your life. I believe there are periods when you have to be willing to let people help you, and that in time you will find the strength and desire to assume more responsibilities for yourself. There are cycles to this disease, as there are with any chronic illness, and when it's time to move from one phase into another, you'll know it.

But that's not how I saw things then. I was lying in the back of my parents' car—*sitting* for two hours would have been too painful—thinking I would never be an independent woman again. When my doctor "sentenced" me to Daniel Freeman, it was for three weeks (okay, so it wound up being more than twelve, but I knew that I would eventually be released), but now there was no light at the end of the tunnel. I had no idea how long I would have to stay with my parents. To be honest, I left the hospital with the mind-set that I would probably be dependent on my parents for the rest of my life.

When we arrived in Bakersfield and drove up our steep driveway, I felt a sense of relief. Dad set up my wheelchair and pushed me up to the front door. It was such a welcome sight! The level of familiarity, the warmth and comfort that seemed to resonate from the walls themselves . . . I felt just like a kid again. Inside, though, things were different. Dad pushed me up to the kitchen table, and as he and my mother unloaded the car, I looked around and noticed the floors. My goodness! The beautiful carpet that my parents loved so much was gone. Not gone, really, but hidden. Dad had taken it upon himself to lay plywood throughout the house so that I could maneuver my wheelchair more easily. In the bathroom he had installed metal bars in the shower stall, to make it easier for me to bathe. Again, there was no discussion about any of this. My parents just did it. They went to enormous effort to adapt their home to my needs, to make it possible for me to live with them again.

When Dad returned to the kitchen he asked, "Well, what do you think?"

I blinked back the tears. "I think it looks great, Dad. Thanks." He bent over so that I could give him a big hug. What made this gesture even more impressive was the fact that my parents didn't have a lot of money in those days, so Dad did the work himself, with his own hands. The job had been done carefully, expertly, and with love.

"Come on," he said. "It's already been a long day. Let's get you into bed."

Life in my Bakersfield cocoon (as I came to think of it) was certainly comfortable enough; Mom and Dad catered to my every need, and it was nice to reclaim a sense of privacy that I

couldn't have at Daniel Freeman. But with that privacy came loneliness. For the most part, I was confined to the house. Once a week
one of my parents would drive me to Los Angeles so that I could
visit my doctor, have blood drawn, and get physical therapy. Because L.A. was two hours away, this was an all-day affair. If it represented a monumental inconvenience for my parents, it was nothing
less than the highlight of the week for me; it was a break from the
boredom and routine of shuffling and wheeling around my house.

My family lived on a hillside above Bakersfield Junior College,
site of the only bell tower in town. I grew up listening to those
chimes, and I had always loved their sound, the way they echoed so
beautifully across the hills. The chimes at Bakersfield Junior College
rang promptly at five minutes before eight each morning, supposedly as a signal to the townspeople that it was time to get up and get
moving; time for school or work; time to get on with the business of
life. Quite often those chimes would serve as my alarm clock. But a
weird thing happened: instead of eliciting a smile, as they routinely
did when I was a girl, the chimes made me sad. To the rest of Bakersfield, the bell tower was a pleasant reminder that another day was
about to begin, a day filled with hope and promise, with opportunity. For me it signaled nothing more than the passing of time.
Twenty-four more hours of pain, boredom, restlessness. It was a
vivid, almost palpable, reminder that I was stuck at home, and that
my only job was to make the transition from bed to wheelchair to
bathroom to kitchen . . . and back to bed. It took more than two
hours for this seventy-nine-pound weakling to get ready to face the
day; it wasn't unusual for me to be pouring a bowl of cereal at just
about the time the rest of Bakersfield was getting ready for lunch.

The bell chimes became a daily reminder that life was passing me
by, and before long I sank into a depression. I felt sorry for myself.
Worst of all, I experienced a deep crisis of faith. All this was predictable—it's a pattern that is likely to be experienced by anyone

who is battling a chronic illness—but I hadn't anticipated it. I thought I would be happy at home. Instead, I reached a depth of sadness that in many ways exceeded even what I had felt in the hospital. I found myself questioning my relationship with God. I had always been a believer in God; I had always found strength and solace in religion and faith. Now, though, I felt abandoned, angry. On more than one occasion I found myself asking, *Why are you doing this to me? What did I do to deserve it?* There were no answers, of course, but I manufactured them anyway. Maybe God was punishing me for that piece of bubble gum I had taken off the counter without paying for it when I was five years old. Maybe it was payback for sampling my father's cigarettes. There had to be an answer!

But there wasn't. I was searching for logic and reason and order in a disease that is patently illogical. I went through a period of time when I hated God, when I blamed Him for everything that had happened to me, for all my suffering and pain. This was ridiculous, but it was also the only way I could make any sense out of what was happening. I have since come to realize these are stages that you have to work through, and that everyone deals with chronic pain and illness in his or her own time and manner. It's a long war, and battles will be won and lost along the way. Blaming God for your circumstances is merely one way of trying to find a path out of the darkness. It's trying to find a spot in your mind where you can begin to take control of the situation, or at least some part of the situation. Lashing out at God, rejecting religion, in the short term, helped me find a measure of peace. I had someone to blame, somewhere to direct all the bad feelings inside me. But my anger toward God was only temporary. After a few months I stopped asking, "Why am I in this position?" and began asking, "How do I get *out* of this position?"

You find out who you are at a time like this. You reach deep inside and find reserves you never knew existed. One of the ways you do this is by going back to your childhood and examining who you really are at your core. You know: *What did Mom and Dad teach me?*

How did I look at the world? I knew I was a good and decent person. I didn't cheat people. I always looked for the best in people. I was someone who worked hard and did well in school. I was someone utterly and completely in love with life. But now here I was, a miserable, self-pitying wretch. I was basically wasting my life, and I wasn't even thirty years old.

So I gave myself a kick in the butt. Not right away, obviously. These transformations rarely occur overnight (except in the movies), but with diligence and perseverance, and a good deal of help from others, I pulled myself out of a very deep and profound funk. Before long the chimes of Bakersfield Junior College no longer sang, "Woe is me." Instead, they became my personal call to action: "Get up, Amye! Get going! You have work to do, girl!"

The first step was to create a dialogue. I would make "to-do" lists each night, so that the next day would be filled with activity of one sort or another. I would carry on conversations with myself, literally sit in my room and say:

"What's up tomorrow, Amye?"

"We're gonna get showered, dressed, and then we're going to the library to do some work. It's time to plan a strategy for minimizing the effects of this blasted disease. You on board?"

"Absolutely. Can't wait!"

Arthritis had taken huge chunks of my body, but it hadn't taken my mind. In my head I was still a go-getter, and there was no reason for that to change. So I asked my mother to begin driving me to the library on a regular basis. In those days, unfortunately, the Internet was only a gleam in the young entrepreneurial eyes of Bill Gates and his buddies. Home-based research, which has become so much more accessible in the twenty-first century, was little more than a dream. But I had the local library, and it soon became my home away from home. There I began to read about arthritis, devouring every volume I could find. Most of the books, to be perfectly honest, were completely meaningless to me. The author would write some-

thing like "Arthritis may be crippling . . ." or "Arthritis may be painful
. . ." and I'd take the book, slam it closed, and laugh out loud: "*May
be?* It is crippling. And it is obviously painful. Come on, people!"

These books just weren't relevant to me. I was looking for advice
and wisdom on how to handle the *emotional* component of arthritis.
I eventually found some information in books about spirituality,
motivation, pain management, positive mental attitude, meditation.
Books by Norman Vincent Peale, for example, and Dr. David Byrne,
a wonderful professor who specializes in mood therapy. One of the
books that had the most profound effect on me was a cancer handbook titled *Getting Well Again*, by O. Carl Simonton, M.D. Rather
than detailing the physical horrors and medical options of cancer
therapy, this was a thoughtful rumination on the emotional side of
cancer. Among other things, it offered the reader strategies for
beating back the disease and coping with pain through various vi-
sualization techniques. Well, it wasn't a great leap for me to apply
these techniques to my own situation. Like the cancer patient, I
was fighting not only for my life but also for the quality of my life,
and I needed every weapon I could get. So I took this model from
cancer and applied it to my arthritis. I'd close my eyes and envision
a giant video game inside my body, my own Pac-Man. The "good"
cells would rush about my body, devouring all the "bad" cells.
Whether this was an appropriate or accurate image didn't really
matter—it worked for me. Psychologically and emotionally, I felt
an almost immediate improvement.

Fate took me further in this direction when I was reading the *Los
Angeles Times* one morning and spotted an advertisement in which
Dr. Simonton's name was prominently featured. It turned out he
was going to be teaching a class at the Ambassador Hotel in L.A.,
one day a week for six weeks. Without hesitation I picked up the
telephone and called the number in the advertisement. I explained
to the woman who answered that I did not have cancer, but that I
was suffering from severe rheumatoid arthritis (I'd never just

blurted it out like that before), and I respected and admired Dr. Simonton, and really wanted to attend his class.

The woman was polite, but resolute. "I'm sorry. There are only twenty spots available, and we're reserving them all for cancer patients."

"Please," I implored. "I've been reading the book and I've gotten a lot out of it. It would mean so much to me to be part of this class."

"Well . . ."

"Look," I interrupted. "Let me tell you who I am." I proceeded to tell this woman, this stranger, the whole Amye Leong story. Apparently, she was moved, or at least impressed by my determination, because I was offered a spot in Dr. Simonton's class. The trips to Los Angeles became even more hectic, because they now included a three-hour class in the afternoon, along with visits to my rheumatologist and physical therapy sessions. The schedule was exhausting but the benefits were enormous, because this class helped me so much. I learned how to meditate, to visualize, to relax. I learned how to imagine writing the word RELAX with the index finger of one hand in the palm of the other, in such a way that by the time I was through writing, my entire body would feel relaxed. Granted, it took me about an hour to do this the first time I tried, but by the end of the course I had it down to a matter of minutes. Maybe most important of all, I learned how to focus—how to *really* focus—on interpreting my pain, on minimizing the pain, on figuring out what I wanted to do with the rest of my life. I learned all over again the importance of setting goals and chasing them vigorously.

When I was released from the hospital, I held only the slimmest of hope that I'd ever get out of a wheelchair, and as the months at my parents' house rolled by, with them taking care of my every need, that flicker of hope was doused. In Dr. Simonton's class the fire was rekindled. I began to visualize myself folding up my wheelchair and putting it in the closet. I saw myself walking without assistance. And slowly that little grain of hope began to grow. Once that image had been crystallized in my mind, there was only one thing left to do (well, that's not quite true, but at least there was a *first* thing to do): plan a course of action.

Confrontation was part of this plan. You have to take responsibility for your own treatment and healing, and to do that you have to be willing to challenge the people who are supposed to be taking care of you. So, on my next visit to the doctor's office I said, "My goal is to get out of this wheelchair. How come you've never asked me about that?"

He seemed surprised. More than that really. He seemed confused, almost as if he hadn't understood the question.

"Amye, my job is to treat you medically and that's what I'm doing."

What an enlightening exchange this turned out to be. It had never occurred to him to inquire about my goals, and it had never occurred to me that he wasn't interested in my goals. Goal setting is the patient's responsibility, and if you want your doctor to be part of a team that helps you achieve those goals, you can't be shy about sharing them. My goal was not to be in a wheelchair for the rest of my life. My goal was not to be on immunosuppressive drugs for the rest of my life. There was a distinct chance that reality would dictate otherwise, but I imagined—I envisioned—a life without wheelchairs and wall-to-wall medications. Once I shared this information with my doctor, he was extremely receptive.

"Okay," he said. "Let's work on it together."

"Great. Now . . . what can we do to get me out of this wheelchair? As quickly as possible?"

He didn't hesitate. "You need surgery, probably a lot of it."

"Fine," I said. "Where do we start?"

He looked at the ground. "At the bottom. With your feet."

At this point I wasn't thinking about a long-term program of surgical management. I was thinking only of taking one step at a time, both literally and metaphorically. So I had both feet surgically reconstructed by Dr. Steven Schwartz, a Los Angeles–based orthopedic surgeon. It was an agonizing and tedious procedure in which my toe joints were fused together with pins and screws. I returned home with tiny metal skewers protruding from my toes and instructions to keep my feet dry at all costs. To allow the feet to get wet was to risk infection, and infection, in someone with an immune system gone berserk, is a very dangerous thing. What the doctors seemed to forget was that I was still an arthritis patient, with numerous joints inflamed and sore. I needed my morning shower to soothe and coax my muscles and joints into facing another day. Thankfully, with the help of garbage bags wrapped around my feet to shield them from the water and the assistance of my mother, I was able to maintain my usual regimen.

As the weeks past, I could feel the healing process taking root. Within four months my feet felt stronger and they looked better. No longer were they deformed, shriveled-up pieces of sausage. *I had toes!* In every way imaginable, I started to feel better. I started standing again, and taking steps in short, turbulent bursts that left me exhausted. I was determined to practice learning to walk all over again. I began using platform crutches, the kind that cradled my elbows to protect my wrists and hands. Eventually, and perhaps inevitably, thoughts of independence flooded my mind.

I needed to be closer to my medical team, and I just knew I had to give my parents their "space." I rented part of a house in Rolling Hills, a breathtakingly beautiful community near Los Angeles. Under normal circumstances it would have been far out of my price range, especially because I had no job and was on disability. But as luck and fate would have it, I wound up in a shared environment, living in part of a house owned by G.P.—my nickname for a quirky and compassionate man.

When I told my parents of my decision, they were surprised, even shocked.

"Who will get your groceries?" my father asked. "Who will drive you to the doctor?" He paused and looked at my mother. "Who will protect you?"

As he talked, my resolve intensified. More than ever I knew that the time had come to strike out on my own—wheelchair, crutches, and all. I haven't the words to adequately profess the love I feel for my parents. They have been there for me through extraordinarily difficult times, and they continue to be at my side today. But it was clear to me then that they had reverted to treating me like a child. For the sake of my own sanity, and the sake of their marriage and privacy, I needed to go.

9

The Bionic Woman

Dr. Schwartz had explained to me that the reconstruction of my feet was merely the first step in a surgical management plan that would take years to complete, but I really hadn't listened to him. I had heard only the word "step," as in "walk." One of the most significant challenges for anyone with arthritis is to avoid the temptation to look for the quick fix. Desperation is common, and understandable, but you have to realize that arthritis management is a lifelong process fueled by hard work, determination, vigilance, and expert medical care. In the early stages of my arthritis I had sought a pharmacological silver bullet; now, from Dr. Schwartz, I wanted a surgical silver bullet.

Fix my feet, get me out of this wheelchair, let me get on with my life!

Rarely, if ever, is the solution so simple. And so it was that nearly six months after having my feet reconstructed, I was back in Dr. Schwartz's office, discussing the next phase of my program. By this time I had come to the realization that orthopedic surgeons would always be important people in my life. When you have chronic arthritis, an orthopedic surgeon is more than just your doctor; he's one of your best friends. Or, at least, he should be, because when you go through joint-replacement or joint-reconstruction surgery, you'll need his help and advice more often than you can imagine. You may have to endure surgery, having prosthetic devices inserted into your body, and most of the time you aren't given a manual. Little information was available when I embarked on my program. No one offered to tell me what to expect two years down the road, let alone five or ten years. It was amazing. When you buy a car, you get a maintenance book with very specific instructions: *Oil change every three thousand miles; transmission service every thirty thousand miles; tune-up at sixty thousand miles.* Nothing like that was available to me when I began my surgical management program in the late '80s. Unless I was deliberate and assertive about seeking advice and information, I remained ignorant.

Fortunately it's very different today. Orthopedic surgeons do routinely educate their patients about what to expect from surgery, and how to maximize the results through rehabilitation and post-operative examinations. They may tell the patient, "We'll be seeing you regularly for the first six months, and we'll be doing X rays every year thereafter." And there are many other resources besides your surgeon, including information from the American Academy of Orthopaedic Surgeons and other reliable websites. But in the '80s, many physicians routinely did the work and just moved on. You'd get an artificial joint, a pat on the back, and never hear from them again, which was a very frightening thing. I wanted a buyer's guide for every single joint replacement, and none existed.

It was my good fortune to have as a teammate Dr. Schwartz, who was not only a talented surgeon but also an honest man, knowledgeable about the medical fraternity. In explicit language he told me exactly what I would have to do to walk, use my arms, and reclaim some semblance of the life I once knew. He told me they could rebuild me. They had the technology. If I was willing, if I had the strength and courage, they could transform me from the wheelchair into a real-life version of the Bionic Woman.

There was just one caveat.

"I can't do it," he said.

"Why not?"

"Because I'm not a specialist. You need to see the people who are the very best in their field. You need to see the best knee doctor for your knees, the best shoulder doctor for your shoulders, the best hand doctor for your hands."

That sounded complicated, but it also made sense.

"There's one other problem," Dr. Schwartz went on. "You're going to have trouble convincing these people to work on you."

"Why?"

"Because you're not a prime candidate."

This sounded ludicrous. "What do you mean? I'm in a wheelchair."

"I know," he said, nodding. "But you're too young. Any doctor who does a joint replacement on you is practically guaranteeing himself a bad result. You have to understand, the goal is to make sure you go to the grave with that joint replacement intact. If you outlast the prosthesis, the doctor's reputation is tarnished, and he looks bad."

He paused and smiled. "No one wants to look bad."

Fortunately, the very thing that would dissuade some surgeons from working on me would also prove to be an enticement to the cream of the crop. The '80s was a frontier time for joint replacement or arthroplasty surgeries. Because the technology was not as enlightened as it is today, surgical success was heavily dependent on the ideal candidate for this procedure. Young, active types (even if it was only a dream to me at the time) with severe RA were certainly not considered ideal candidates. But I was determined to get out of the wheelchair and return to a productive life.

In the past sixteen years I've been hospitalized seventeen times and had sixteen different surgical procedures, including twelve joint replacements. Surgical management is today considered an acceptable, if last-resort, approach to treating severe arthritis. At the time that I met with Dr. Schwartz, no one had ever heard of anyone being rebuilt from the bottom up in this manner. It just didn't happen. And the very fact that it hadn't happened was precisely the right carrot to dangle in front of a hotshot orthopedic surgeon.

But how do you find the very best physicians? You can't just go on the Internet and do a search—in 1985 you couldn't, anyway. Today, although its easy to search the Internet, care must be taken in finding reliable and credible information. There are different motives and criteria for declaring someone "the best." So, understanding what my needs were, and how I was going to select the right person, I began the process of searching for a knee surgeon (we wanted to do my knees next, because they were the most heavily damaged joints). This meant asking a lot of questions. I started with my friend Tina; as a physical therapist in the Los Angeles area, she had worked with patients referred by some of the most accomplished orthopedic surgeons in the country. I also queried my rheumatologist, my two physician uncles, and any number of friends and acquaintances I had met during the course of my treatment. I started reading books and magazines. If I discovered someone who had undergone a knee replacement, I didn't hesitate to reach out to that person for a firsthand account of the experience.

The most important thing you can do if you're contemplating a joint replacement (or any other type of treatment for your arthritis) is to find reliable sources of information. You can start with the Arthritis Foundation, a U.S. nonprofit organization whose mission is to improve lives through leadership in the prevention, control, and cure of arthritis and related diseases. The Arthritis Foundation has a primary agenda: to be an advocate for the patient. It will give you reliable information about top-quality care, physicians, therapists, and support groups. Through the Arthritis Foundation's support and education and exercise programs, you'll have access to a vast network of people experienced with the disease, many of them patients who have firsthand, experiential knowledge of your situation and symptoms. I strongly recommend that you reach out. Not only will you become educated and enlightened; you'll also connect on an intensely personal level. In my search, I spoke with other patients to get their opinions about physicians, but I also wanted to ask them, in very specific terms, exactly what to expect from the surgery. How much did it hurt? How long were they in the hospital? When were they able to walk? Doctors have a set of answers for questions such as these, but they can differ markedly from the answers provided by patients. Information provided by patients is purely experiential and can complement what is provided by the doctor.

After talking with literally dozens of people, I ended up selecting an orthopedic surgeon named Lawrence Dorr. Dr. Dorr was an esteemed knee specialist in Los Angeles and one of the world's foremost orthopedic surgeons. An entire floor of Centinela Hospital in Los Angeles was devoted to patients of Dr. Dorr, and their numbers routinely included professional athletes and entertainers. An air of professionalism and confidence permeated the whole floor. It was like an expertly managed factory, with every nurse and rehabilitation specialist thoroughly schooled in the Dorr surgical protocol.

I was impressed with the results achieved by Dr. Dorr and his colleagues, and I was reasonably confident in their hands. I wanted a master technician, and that's what I had found. Before you decide to have joint-replacement surgery, however, you should understand something very important: The surgeon alone cannot dictate success. In my opinion, joint-replacement surgery is a sixty-forty deal: 40 percent of the responsibility for achieving a positive result falls on the shoulders of the doctor; the remaining 60 percent falls on the patient. Does that sound hard to believe? Think about it. That doctor will be working on you for two or three hours, but you'll be living with the prosthesis for the rest of your life. You'll visit his office regularly at first (and then periodically), and you'll have an opportunity to ask questions, but make no mistake: you are the one who will have to drive the rehabilitation. You'll have to persevere through countless exercises on days when you're exhausted and sore. You'll have to motivate yourself to move beyond your fear of pain. You'll have to monitor your progress and be an advocate for yourself when things seem to be going badly. No one else will do that job for you. It's all up to you.

Joint-replacement surgery is brutal, demanding work, and you want the best set of hands possible putting you back together. Today I have a number of friends who are orthopedic surgeons, and for the life of me I don't know how they can stomach the work. If we're at a dinner party together, I'll tease them by saying something like "How can you possibly eat meat after the kind of day you've had? How can you even look at it?" Usually they'll just laugh and dig in.

Honestly, though, the psyche of an orthopedic surgeon is amazing. So brutal and invasive is the work that a certain distance must be maintained. Think of what you see when you watch a hospital drama on television. The doctor picks up the scalpel, places metal on skin, and then the camera cuts away and your imagination takes over. Well, in real life these guys keep right on going. They cut and twist and pull and sew and they do it two or three times a day. They spend a good portion of their lives wearing masks and gowns. They realize that a human being is connected to that joint, but to a great extent they divorce themselves from this reality. It's a protective mechanism that allows the surgeon to do his job effectively, for to be overly concerned with the patient as a human being, to be preoccupied with her emotional state, is to risk performing at something less than peak efficiency. The surgeon would prefer to think of himself as a master craftsman, maybe even an artist, and the joint as a work of art.

As much as I empathize with the surgeon's need to separate his heart from his hands, I think it's important that he be cognizant of the fact that a joint is more than just bone and sinew and tendons and cartilage. So I repeatedly reminded Larry Dorr that this wasn't just any knee he was fixing—it was Amye Leong's knee. "This knee is going to allow me to walk," I said. "It's going to turn my entire life around." I wanted to make sure he knew the personality behind this piece of flesh he was about to cut into. Fear and naiveté fueled this approach prior to my initial knee surgery, but even as I've become more experienced, more aware of the challenges faced by surgeons and their need to be technicians first, psychologists second, and compassionate humanists third, it has remained a staple of my arsenal in the war against arthritis. Throughout my surgical management program, I made a point of befriending every surgeon who worked on me, and I think that's a sound strategy. There's no doubt that, first and foremost, you want a skilled technician, but once you've identified that person, you must give him a reason to care about you as a person, and not merely as a "procedure." You must find a way to humanize the experience, so he won't forget there is a living, breathing person on that operating table.

You can accomplish this task merely through cooperation, or you can resort to more drastic and comedic measures, as I did a few years later, when I was undergoing surgery on one of my elbows. After I was prepped for surgery, but before I was wheeled into the operating room, I wrote a message to my elbow surgeon, Dr. Roy Meals of UCLA and taped it to my arm. "This is an important elbow," the message read. "I'm going to use this elbow to eat, write, and advocate for other people with arthritis. I just know you'll do a good job!" Well, as it turned out Dr. Meals saw the note just before he leaned into me with a scalpel. He stopped, read the message, and began smiling and chuckling. I later found out that the doctor loved my note and planned to have it framed in his office, where it would serve as a daily reminder of the reason he became a doctor in the first place: to help other people.

During my initial consultation with Dr. Dorr he had made it painfully clear that I would need not just one, but two knee replacements. "Oh yeah," he said after examining the X rays and reviewing my medical history. "You need these and you need them right away. And if it were up to me, I'd do them both at the same time."

Yikes!

That scared me. I suspected I would need to have both knees replaced eventually, but the thought of a bilateral knee replacement was, well . . . terrifying. What would I stand on while the joints were healing? How would I get out of bed or go to the bathroom? Today it's common for people to have bilateral knee replacements, but in the mid '80s it was more the exception. Even if it had been a reasonable option, I'm not sure I would have selected it. Not on my first joint replacement. To be perfectly candid, I was afraid of the process. I had done my research on the subject; I had plowed through books and journals and articles I could barely comprehend at first. It was complicated surgery, and it sounded just horrific: replacing bone and cartilage with metal, sewing up tendons and ligaments, and inserting glue into the whole mess. In one of my early meetings with Dr. Dorr, he explained that a possible problem in joint replacement was, in fact, a loosening of the prosthesis. The cement most commonly employed in joint-replacement surgery was a close relative of the material used by dentists.

Oh, that's wonderful, I thought. *How often do fillings fall out? All the time!*

Suddenly this didn't seem like such a good idea. I felt a wave of panic rush over me.

Oh, my God! What am I doing here? This is not reliable stuff, and these people don't know what they're doing!

I was tempted to bolt for the door (actually, in my case, I would have *limped* for the door), but something held me back. Intimidating as the surgery might have been, at least it presented the possibility for a better life. It was, in fact, my only hope.

"Okay," I said. "But I can't handle doing both knees at once. Which one do we do first?"

"The destruction in the right knee is more pronounced," Dr. Dorr explained. "Let's start with that one."

He advised me to go home and think about it, to make sure that I was totally committed not only to the surgery but also to the long and arduous rehabilitation that would follow. Three weeks later, after many more trips to the library and countless calls to other surgeons and therapists and anyone else who could provide me with information, I made a decision: I would have the surgery. I called Dr. Dorr's office and set up an appointment for a new knee. The first surgical opening on Dr. Dorr's calendar was two months away, and I used that time to prepare myself not just physically, but mentally and spiritually, for what I suspected would be one of the biggest challenges of my life.

In truth, I really didn't know what to expect, but I knew I had to buy into it. I had to invest myself, heart and soul. (Today we know from studies released by the National Institutes of Health's Office of Alternative Medicine that your belief system can dramatically affect how your body reacts to anything.) I decided to take ownership of this surgery. I bombarded Dr. Dorr with questions, just as I had bombarded other patients. I asked him a thousand questions, and he gave me a thousand and one answers. Without fear I asked him what might seem the silliest questions, but they were important to me.

"You're putting metal in my body—will I weigh more?"

"Is this going to make me feel like I have a foreign part in my body?"

"When I wake up from surgery, how will I feel?"

Dr. Dorr gave me answers without hesitation. They didn't always match the information I had received from others, but they helped me form a broad base of knowledge. By the time I entered the hospital, I felt as though I was as prepared as I could be.

I also felt pretty sick, because, as advised, I had to go off all medication prior to surgery. Some medications for arthritis suppress the immune system. That's good when you're fighting arthritis, but bad when you're recovering from surgery and need your immune system at full strength to ward off infection. So, as advised, I went off everything cold turkey. In the days leading up to my first knee surgery I came to the conclusion that Amye *au natural* is a very sickly individual. I was in such an arthritis flare that I could barely move; I was basically bed-bound, totally reliant once again on the care and assistance of family and friends. Without my usual cocktail of arthritis medications, I was helpless. It made me realize how fortunate I was to have been born in the latter half of the twentieth century, when at least there was reasonably effective medication for people with arthritis.

The return of this incessant, excruciating pain was discouraging; at the same time, it motivated me by reminding me of just how badly I wanted to be cured . . . or at least repaired. What I endured in preparation for joint-replacement surgery was pure agony, but if the outcome was freedom from a wheelchair, then it was worth it. In a weird twist of fate, the pain of knee-replacement surgery turned out to be less than I had anticipated, mainly because I experienced an intense flare in my other joints while I was undergoing surgery. When I awoke in the recovery room, and in the days afterward, I felt more pain in my elbows, hands, and shoulders than I did in my new knee.

What was supposed to be a seven-day hospitalization became three and a half weeks. While postoperative recovery was progressing for my knee, the rest of me was suffering from a worsening arthritis flare. In that time I learned a great deal about myself and the importance of having a positive mental attitude. The ability to create calmness in a chaotic situation, the ability to control your pain despite your natural tendency to panic . . . those are skills of immeasurable value. I've discovered that when there is an emergency, people usually react in one of two ways: They either panic or they experience a clarity that allows them to go immediately and effectively into action. Arthritis is a disease that requires clarity. Panic will only make it worse.

How do you achieve clarity? It's different for each person. For me, it's about taking a deep breath, letting go of my fear, and focusing on the real issues. Being wheeled on a gurney into an operating room before surgery is an experience that can cause almost anyone to panic. Even after having done it sixteen times, I still feel the anxiety bubbling up through my body. In this case, I focus. I focus on the faces of the nurses, anesthesiologist, and others who are part of the operating room. I focus on why I decided to go with that particular surgeon for this operation and recall his competence and the sense of trust we were able to establish with each other. And I focus on my breathing, trying to slow it down but taking deep breaths. Most important of all, I see in my mind's eye the surgery going perfectly and my body healing exceptionally well. In other words, I visualize and meditate and pray . . . and I always feel better because of this.

As important as it is to prepare prior to surgery, I knew the real work would begin the moment I awoke. It would take days, weeks, and maybe months for tissues to heal; and it was my responsibility to be a full participant in my recovery and rehabilitation. With every in-hospital instruction about physical therapy, rest, and nutrition, I became a willing and eager partner. I was captain of my own destiny at that point. Whether I would be able to move that joint to its full range successfully would depend upon my commitment during rehabilitation. And I was extremely committed and motivated. My wheelchair had a funny way of motivating me!

But the real test for me was rehabilitation in my home setting. It is so easy *not* to do exercises. There are a million excuses: I hurt too much today; I'm too tired; I don't want to upset my incisions. The list goes on and on! But I learned that these kinds of excuses can make the difference between getting a mediocre result or an excellent result from surgery. If I was going through all the trouble, pain, disruption, and expense of having the surgery, then I wanted to have the best opportunity for a positive result. So I took on at-home rehabilitation like a job—a new and important job. I evaluated myself at the end of each week to see if I was being a good employee and doing what was expected. Did I go out of my way to do more? Was I attentive to my body, proactive in my wound care and physical therapy? My physical rehabilitation was a business, and I decided to give it the proper attention.

More than four months passed before I realized something was missing in my life, and what was missing was the relentless presence of pain I had been experiencing for years in my right knee. It took that long for my body to recover from the shock of surgery and the various flares caused by my withdrawal from medication. Once the realization settled in, though, I was practically gleeful.

Wow! It worked!

That was my initial reaction. My second reaction was *Why did I wait so long?* And my third reaction was *Let's do the other one!*

Six months after I left Centinela Hospital with a new right knee, I returned for a second knee replacement. I was much more confident this time around. I was on a first-name basis with most of the nurses and therapists, and I was thoroughly schooled in the Dr. Dorr routine. Most important of all, I knew my surgeon would do the job well. Unlike the first surgery, I did not have to contend with a fear of the unknown. I knew precisely what to expect. The procedure would still be awful, the recovery traumatic and painful, but it was far less frightening and mysterious. Having a sense of what to expect when you're entering a hospital is important. If you're about to experience a procedure for the first time, seek out someone who has been through it. Consult with your doctor or physical therapist to get the names of others who have gone through a similar procedure. Check local arthritis support groups and on-line chat groups from reputable websites. Arm yourself with information. Otherwise, you may find that the anxiety is worse than the procedure itself.

Unfortunately, although the surgery went smoothly enough, recovery from my second knee replacement proved to be a bit complicated. I lost a lot of blood during the operation and needed a blood transfusion. The next day, while sitting up in bed in my private room (the weakened state of my immune system made it unwise for me to have a roommate) having a conversation with my father, I felt my body temperature suddenly drop.

"Dad," I said, "I'm really cold."

My father stood up, walked to the closet, and retrieved an extra blanket. As he leaned over me, the room began to spin, just as it had when I went into shock following plasmapheresis several years earlier. Just before everything went black I could hear my father screaming, "Nurse! Nurse!"

When I regained consciousness a nurse was sitting at the end of my bed holding my hand. My dad was sitting in a chair, his face contorted with worry, his complexion a ghastly white. There was a doctor standing over me, smiling.

"Welcome back, Amye," he said, as though I had just taken a little walk down to the corner store.

"What happened?"

"Well, we had a little reaction to the blood," he said.

We? We didn't have anything. I had it!

Blood transfusions seem like such a normal part of the surgical experience, but they can be problematic. The body can reject blood just as it rejects any foreign substance, and having a weakened immune system only complicates matters and increases the likelihood of postsurgical problems. Not only that, but blood screening in the 1980s was a far less comprehensive process than it is today. Three years after my second knee replacement I attended a dinner party at the home of my rheumatologist, a delightful and compassionate man named Gideon Darvish. It was a wonderful party with about a dozen guests, including several doctors who had put considerable effort into rebuilding Amye Leong. My relationships with these people had begun in a clinical setting, but had since blossomed into deep friendships. Still, I wasn't quite prepared for what transpired that evening.

At one point, as people were leaning forward, talking across the table, carrying on various conversations, the talk turned to HIV. This, after all, was 1989, and AIDS was an intensely hot topic, especially in the medical community. Dr. C. Everett Koop, the surgeon general, had by now sent out a strong letter of warning to hospitals and physicians all over the world strongly recommending, among other things, screening of all blood to be used in transfusions. Suddenly one of my surgeon friends said, loudly enough for everyone to hear, "You know, Amye, you're not out of the woods yet."

"Excuse me?"

"That transfusion we gave you back in 'eighty-five? You have another year to go before you're safe."

I just stared at him. By now the whole room had fallen silent. A few people nodded, and then the conversation turned to other topics.

Well, thank you very much, Doc, for letting ten other people—including my boyfriend!—know that I might possibly have contracted HIV through tainted blood. Anything else we'd like to share?

He had intended no harm. We were all friends, and to members of the medical fraternity such talk was considered normal and appropriate fodder for dinner-table conversation. But I would have preferred that he told me in private. Maybe it was no big deal to anyone else, but it was a big deal to me. To be honest, I hadn't even thought about the possibility that I had contracted HIV and the virus had been lying dormant in my body, waiting for the right moment to come to life. I assumed that enough time had passed and that I had dodged a bullet. Now I was being told that I had another year to sweat it out, and I was being given this disturbing news in a very public setting. It was a sobering reminder that although I was a frequent guest at the medical country club, I was not, and never would be, a member. I looked at things differently, and I always would.

Within a few weeks after my second knee surgery, I began taking daily walks in a nearby park. My gait was stilted and awkward at first—it had been such a long time since I'd walked normally and without pain that I'd almost forgotten how it was done—but I could not have been happier. So impressive were the results, so immediate and pronounced the improvement, that I couldn't wait to continue with the surgical program. Dr. Dorr's work on my knees had convinced me that I was finally on the road to recovery, and I wanted to sustain the momentum. Even as I sweated through the arduous process of knee rehabilitation, I began searching for the right person to work on the next set of joints that would need replacement: my shoulders.

Shoulder replacements then were rare; only a handful of U.S. orthopedic surgeons were even attempting them, and more often than not the results were not encouraging. The shoulder is a smaller, more complicated joint, and thus more challenging from a surgical standpoint. Nevertheless, I was resolute in my decision to have the work done. As was the case with my knees, I really saw no alternative. My shoulders had deteriorated to the point where I could barely move my arms. My elbows were always bent at my waist, sort of hooked into my belt, in an effort to take the pressure off my shoulders, giving me the short-armed appearance of a smallish tyrannosaurus rex, albeit a rather benign one. Eating was a laborious and painful process in which I had to bring my head down to my hands, and sometimes my plate. On the worst of days it felt as though my shoulders would simply fall out of their sockets and my arms would drop to the floor.

Unable to face the prospect of living that way any longer, I went to New York to meet with Dr. Charles Neer, an orthopedic surgeon affiliated with Columbia Presbyterian Hospital. Dr. Neer was known to be the world's best "shoulder man," and in our initial consultation he certainly seemed comfortable with that unofficial title.

"Yeah, you need this surgery, and I'm the surgeon to do it," he said. More than just confident, he exuded cockiness, even arrogance, which didn't bother me in the least. This was complicated stuff (even after reading dozens of articles and having my friend Tina translate the medical jargon, I still wasn't sure how the procedure would work), and I wanted a surgeon who was utterly free of self-doubt performing the work. I wanted someone who was absolutely certain the result would be positive, and Dr. Neer sure seemed to be that person.

One of the things I discovered when I returned to New York a few weeks later was that there wasn't necessarily a correlation between the talent of the doctor and the aesthetic quality of the hospital in which he practiced medicine. Indeed, walking into Columbia Presbyterian Hospital was an enlightening and disturbing experience, a real window into the world of big-city health care, and how it differs from one metropolitan area to another. I had been accustomed to beautiful Centinela Hospital in Los Angeles, with its glistening windows, spotless rooms, and antibacterial airflow to prevent in-

fection. At Columbia Presbyterian I was assigned to a room supposedly reserved for "good" patients (translation: those who have
reliable insurance or are otherwise capable of paying for the room),
and yet, when I was wheeled into my room I was appalled by what I
saw. It was dark and dank. The bed was one of those crank-up models, like something out of the 1930s. Near the bed was an old desk
with the varnish rubbed off and a lamp that was notable only for its
yellowed and dented lampshade, on which someone appeared to
have urinated. As for the view, well, I'm not sure, because the windows looked as if they hadn't been cleaned in the previous decade.
Overall, it reminded me of a motel in one of L.A.'s sleazier neighborhoods.

"Stop!" I said.

The nurse who was accompanying us seemed surprised by my reaction. "What's wrong?"

"This can't be my room," I said.

She shrugged. "Yes, it is."

"What am I paying for here?"

"You're paying for a room, a bed, and basic nursing care." She
looked around the room, clearly annoyed by my insolence. "And
that's what you're getting."

The most basic nursing care, I learned, did not include a nurse
who would come running into my room each time I buzzed, as it did
at Centinela. If I wanted that degree of attention, I would have to
hire a private-duty nurse at a cost of nearly a thousand dollars per
day! My father and I talked it over briefly and agreed to spring for
the private nurse; with any luck, my insurance company would re-
imburse me later. And so, for the next thirty-three days, twenty-four
hours a day, I shared my awful little room with a dour-faced private
nurse. She did her job and she did it well, but clearly companionship and conversation were not part of the package.

Did I mention that my stay at Columbia Presbyterian lasted
thirty-three days? Yes, I did. What I didn't say was that it was sup-

posed to last seven to ten days. While the shoulder replacement it-self went quite well (Dr. Neer was every bit as gifted as I had been led to believe he was), the recovery hit something of a snag. Four days after surgery, with bandages and gauze covering my neck, shoulder, and torso, and still in excruciating pain, I was neither sleeping nor eating. I was beyond grouchy—I was ready to kill someone . . . or die trying. Now, this was not my typical reaction to surgery. Granted, I was unhappy with the surroundings and the at-titude of some of the staff, but by now I took pride in my ability to endure the pain of arthritis and all its various treatments with a healthy combination of grit and humor. Something about this was unusual. The pain was like nothing I'd ever experienced. It was re-lentless. It was . . . *different.*

Finally, on the fifth day, at about three-thirty in the morning, I succumbed to the pain and the sleeplessness and the hunger. I lashed out with all the anger and energy I could muster:

"Nurse!" I screamed. "Get a doctor!"

The nurse calmly tried to take my hand. "Amye, you've already had a pain shot. I can't give you another one for three more—"

I cut her off. "I don't want a shot! I want a doctor! Something's wrong here!"

Never had I been so belligerent. But it wasn't just madness at work. I had been through two knee replacements, and I was fully aware of that joint's capacity for inflicting pain on its host. Shoul-der surgery was supposed to be no worse. Either I had softened in the intervening months or something terrible was happening. I chose to believe the latter.

A few minutes later a disheveled young man stumbled into the room. His hair was matted, his eyes bloodshot, his white coat turned nearly inside out. His entire look fairly screamed: *Intern on call!*

"What's the problem?" he asked, politely enough.

I took a deep breath, swallowed some of the pain that was now racking my upper body. "Please," I began, "you have to help me. I've been through joint replacements in the past. I shouldn't be in this kind of pain four days after surgery. I feel like I'm on fire. My arms . . . my chest . . . my whole back. What's going on?"

"Okay," he said. "Try to stay calm. Let's take a look."

With that he began to unravel the gauze, as if I were a mummy or something. As the layers fell away and my skin became visible, I noticed his eyes widening. All of a sudden he didn't look like a physician; he looked like a scared kid.

"Uh-oh!" he exclaimed. "We've got a problem here."

Not exactly words to inspire confidence, and when I looked down at the gauze, which was now covered with decaying skin, I understood his concern.

"*Ummmm* . . . is that mine?"

He nodded.

I felt like I was going to faint.

"Let's wrap you up," the intern said. "Dr. Neer will be in at five-thirty—that's only a couple of hours from now. I'll make sure he comes right in to see you first, before he starts rounds."

Sure enough, Dr. Neer walked in at five-thirty, trailed by three of his assistants—a trio of young residents presumably handpicked for a prestigeous apprenticeship at the knee of the master. As far as I could tell, they were never allowed to speak until Dr. Neer asked them a question. I got to know these young men during my stay at Columbia, and I came to like them immensely. I also took great pleasure in teasing them about the subservient nature of their jobs. In fact, I liked to call them Charlie Neer and the Neerettes. Sort of like Gladys Knight in the Pips. Dr. Neer was the star, and the Neerettes, simply by virtue of their presence—always a few feet behind—amplified his stardom. Oddly enough, a few years later, at a support group meeting in West Los Angeles, I was approached by a young woman who said, "You know, my brother is an orthopedic resident in New York, and he and the other members of his team called themselves the Neerettes. They said there was a young Chinese woman who had been a patient some time earlier and she had come up with the name. That was you, wasn't it? You're the woman who invented the Neerettes!" So it was still going on, after all those years. The cast of the Neerettes changed regularly, but the name lived on! I couldn't believe it and chuckled proudly.

Anyway, Dr. Neer proceeded to remove my bandages, just as the young intern had earlier. Once again, I sat there helplessly, naked from the waist up, as their eyes practically popped out of their heads. I wouldn't have minded if their reaction stemmed from some great appreciation of my breasts; after all, it had been a while since I'd thought of myself as a hot chick. Alas, they saw me as hot, all right, but not in the way I had hoped. Instead, they were looking at me as though I were a seared duck or a roasted pig.

"It looks like you've had an allergic reaction to the iodine we used to prep you for surgery," Dr. Neer said.

I was stunned. "That was five days ago!"

He nodded grimly. "I know."

Okay, so I wasn't crazy. The pain I'd been experiencing was caused by second-degree burns all over my back, neck, and shoulders. For the past four days my skin had been broiling—the unfortunate, and completely unforseen, result of a reaction to a substance I had tolerated without incident in the past. Who would have guessed? That was another fringe benefit of rheumatoid arthritis: a change in body chemistry. All the surgery and medication had wreaked havoc on my system, rendering me susceptible to all sorts of new illnesses and allergies.

From that point on I was treated as a burn victim. All visitors to my room were required to wear masks. Sterile cloths covered with salve were placed on my body with tweezers and changed every few hours, a process accompanied by no small amount of discomfort. My shoulder rehabilitation, of course, was delayed for several weeks because it was far more important to heal the burns first, especially with my chronically weak immune system. To put it mildly, I was in a bad way. I had traveled all the way across the country to work with a top orthopedic surgeon, and I ended up with burns all over my chest, wondering not only whether the shoulder surgery would be a success but also whether the price would include disfiguring scars over my upper body.

The concern was legitimate. I wore turtlenecks for the better part of the next two years as my skin attempted to heal itself. In time, though, the scars faded. For all my complaining about the unpleasant appearance of Columbia Presbyterian Hospital, and my bad luck with iodine, it became apparent in my recovery that the staff there was every bit as talented and committed as their reputations indicated. Once diagnosed, my burns were treated swiftly and aggressively, which gave me the best shot at a full recovery. My new shoulder was starting to show great promise of movement, as Dr. Neer had said it would. For the first time in many years I could raise my arm shoulder-high.

Dr. Neer was an intensely serious man who never smiled. One day, when I asked him why, he answered with a terse "Because there's nothing to smile about; this is serious business." Toward the end of my hospitalization, I began to tease him.

"Charlie, on the day I leave, I'm gonna get a big smile out of you."

"*Harumph,*" he'd say with a scowl, and then walk away.

When that day came, I was picked up by a limo (I'd made the arrangements myself). As I was saying good-bye to Dr. Neer, I gave him a big kiss on the cheek. He flushed red at first, and then a wide smile crossed his face. I smiled back and waved an index finger at him.

"Told you so!"

I had five hours to kill before catching my plane to Los Angeles, so the limo driver, whose name was Carl, asked me what I'd like to do.

I thought about it for a moment. I'd been in New York for thirty-three days, more than a month in one of the greatest cities on the planet, and virtually every second of that time had been spent in a hospital. Now I had five hours to have some fun. There was only one thing to do.

"Actually," I said, "I'd like to go shopping."

"Okay," he said with a laugh. "I'll tell you what we're going to do. We'll have some lunch, then we'll go to SoHo. And you'll be my princess for the day. I'll hold the doors for you, and you order me around. I don't want you lifting a finger."

Pretty tacky, huh? But you know what? It was one of the most outrageously enjoyable afternoons of my life. We arrived at a funky boutique in SoHo and parked the white stretch limousine right in front. Then Carl, who was a very big, strong guy, opened the door for me with an exaggerated bow at the waist. I slowly got out and shuffled toward the front door of the boutique, which he also opened. Inside, everyone stopped and stared. Here I was, this tiny woman with bandages all over her upper body, with gloves protecting her hands, looking for all the world like the victim of a car bombing or something, accompanied by a mountainous man in a three-piece uniform and a tidy little white cap.

"May we help you?" one of the clerks said to me.

"No, thank you . . . my friend here will take care of everything." I gestured toward Carl, who nodded obediently.

For the next half hour we plowed through rack after rack of clothing. My "butler" would remove a garment, hold it up for my inspection, and I would either approve with a nod, or, more likely, dismiss it with a sniff. After much theater, I settled on an outfit, paid for it, and left the store. Carl carried my package, opened the doors, and helped me into the car. As a crowd of curious shoppers looked on, we drove away, laughing so hard we could barely talk.

"Thank you," I finally said, when I could catch my breath. "You have no idea what that did for my ego."

Carl looked in the rearview mirror and nodded. "My pleasure, ma'am."

10

Found: A New Kind of Family

Advocacy has been a driving force in my life for a long time now. I've had more than my fair share of battles with arthritis, and if there is anything I can do to help others who have been similarly challenged, then I feel I have an obligation to do it. In all candor, though, I must admit that my work grew out of a very personal, even selfish, motivating force.

Prior to my three-month stay at Daniel Freeman Hospital in the 1980s, I had never fully acknowledged or confronted the depth of my illness. While there, I first discovered the importance of education, of understanding my disease in all its myriad forms. And it was there, while sharing brown-bag lunches with my therapists and nurses, that I began to understand the value of exchanging knowledge with people my own age. These people helped me understand arthritis from a professional standpoint, but they could not relate to what was important to me as a young person. Still, I sensed something was missing. In group therapy sessions I was always the youngest in the room, usually by a good thirty or forty years. While there was undeniable relevance and merit to these sessions, I usually felt somewhat isolated. Similarly, even though I formed lasting friendships with the younger therapists, nurses, and doctors, they couldn't possibly understand what I had been through. Not on a personal level, anyway.

I realized that I needed to talk with other young people like myself. But how to find them? At one point I explained to my friend Tina that in college I had started a crisis intervention hot line, and she said, "That's wonderful. Have you ever thought about reaching out to other young people with arthritis?"

"Well, yes, I have thought about it. In fact, I've been thinking about it a lot lately. There must be other young people somewhere in the world who have arthritis. But I've never met any of them."

That was the absolute truth. In my entire life, I had never met another person my age who had severe, debilitating, chronic arthritis. Through conversations with my doctors, I knew they were out there somewhere, probably hiding their illnesses, denying their condition, just as I had for so many years.

"Look," Tina said, "we can do this together. You're stuck in a hospital bed, so let me be your hands and legs. Just tell me what to do, and I'll be happy to do it for you. But you have to come up with the ideas. This is your show."

So, from a hospital bed at Daniel Freeman Hospital, the idea of a young person's arthritis support group was born. Little did we know that there was nothing like this not only in the city of Los Angeles but also in the entire United States of America. I began by making a call to the Arthritis Foundation. In previous years I had made donations to the Arthritis Foundation, but that was about the extent of my involvement. This was the first time I had ever truly reached out.

A pleasant-sounding woman took my phone call. "Arthritis Foundation. May I help you?"

"Hi, my name is Amye Leong, and I'm interested in getting some information on arthritis as it pertains to young people."

Long pause. "I can send you some brochures if you'd like. What's your address?"

"I appreciate that," I said. "But what I really want is to talk with other young people who have arthritis. Can you point me in the right direction?"

Pause. "I don't believe we know of any young people with arthritis here, but I'll tell you what I can do. If you give me your name and number, and if we hear of someone, we can try to get you two together. How's that?"

"Terrific!" I exclaimed. I was ecstatic. If any organization could find a second needle in the haystack, it was probably the Arthritis Foundation. At the very least, I had reason to hope.

A couple of months passed and there was no word from the Arthritis Foundation, no evidence, as far as I could tell, that another young person with arthritis walked—or limped—on the face of the Earth. During one of my visits to Los Angeles for physical therapy and a doctor's appointment, I attended an arthritis support group session. My father dropped me off, and I wheeled into a room with perhaps thirty people in attendance. Virtually all of them seemed to be at least seventy years of age. Bless their hearts, they were universally delightful and gracious. They stopped their conversation the minute I entered the room and one of them said, "Can we help you, dear?"

"I'm not sure," I said sheepishly. "Is this the arthritis support group?"

"Yes, it is. But are you sure this is what you want?"

Apparently, even in a wheelchair, I didn't look like someone who could possibly have arthritis. "If you're talking about arthritis, then this is where I want to be."

"Okay. Come on in!"

Wheeling across the floor, I thought to myself, *How is this going to be relevant to me?* As it turned out, it really wasn't relevant to my needs. They were wonderful people and they were extremely nice to a young interloper like myself, but they really didn't talk about coping with arthritis. They talked mainly about a white elephant sale they were trying to organize, along with some other social activities. Everything on the agenda was important from the standpoint of people bonding together, especially people who have commonality. But I wanted something else. I wanted *information*, preferably experiential information: *Tell me what you know, tell me what you've learned, because I'm too young to be stuck in a wheelchair from arthritis.* That information was not available in this room.

As disappointing as the experience may have been, it did not sour me on support groups. This one wasn't for me, but it didn't turn me off the concept. I liked the community atmosphere, and I admired the spirit and ambition of the men and women in that room. I just needed a different *type* of support group. I knew, somehow, there had to be help available from people dealing with a situation similar to the one I was facing; however, it did occur to me that the mechanism for bringing us together might not be available. That being the case, perhaps it was time to jump in feetfirst and try to get something going. By the time I got into my dad's car for the long ride back to Bakersfield, I had convinced myself: *Amye, it's time to start your own support group.*

Not long after that (and this was about the same time that the chimes of Bakersfield Junior College were serving as a daily kick in the behind), I made a second call to the Arthritis Foundation, this one much longer and more involved. I introduced myself and explained my background. The woman who answered the phone was, once again, unfailingly polite and appropriately unimpressed. I was no one. Well, that isn't quite true. I was one of the 43 million people in the United States who suffered from some form of arthritis, and that alone made me important in the eyes of the Arthritis Foundation. But I wasn't a celebrity. I was neither rich nor famous. I had no great connections in the business or political worlds. I was just a disembodied voice trying to express an idea, trying to sell someone else on a cause that I believed was worthwhile.

"I'm interested in working with young people who have arthritis," I explained.

"Young, meaning what?"

"I'm not sure. From teens to thirties, forties. Younger than most people envision when they think of arthritis."

That seemed to pique her interest. The Arthritis Foundation vigorously supports its constituency and is refreshingly open to ideas and suggestions, even when presented by newcomers. To my astonishment, she said, "Young lady, if you'd like to start something, then go right ahead. I think it's a great idea. We'll send our program director out to meet with you to discuss the specifics. If we like what we hear, we'll back you one hundred percent."

Over the next six months Tina and I worked feverishly to put together a support group for young people with arthritis. We secured the support of Daniel Freeman Hospital, which offered to provide us with a meeting space and free publicity. We came up with a name for our group: Young at Heart, but then quickly changed it to Young *et* Heart. Why? Because we realized that "Young at Heart" is a very popular Frank Sinatra tune embraced by senior citizens worldwide as a way of saying "I may be aging on the outside, but I'm young on the inside." Our group was something quite different. We were trying to say, "I look like I'm young, but I'm aging on the inside. I'm being eaten alive by something that most people think of as an old person's disease."

So we changed the name, replacing "at" with "et," the French word for *and*. Now the message we were trying to convey was "I'm young . . . and I have heart." We put a public-service announcement in the *Los Angeles Times*, figuring that in a city of 10 million people there had to be at least a few young people under the age of fifty with some form of arthritis that had impacted their lives to such an extent that they would want to reach out to other young people with arthritis.

In the spring of 1984, Young et Heart was born. Our first meeting was held in a community room at Daniel Freeman Hospital at eleven o'clock on a Saturday morning. Out of 10 million people, five showed up. Not 5 million . . . not five thousand . . . not five hundred. *Five.* And two of those people were Tina and I. Nevertheless, it was like a homecoming. Tina and I, of course, had arrived early. Anxious and excited, we had set up the room, put out trays of coffee and cookies, assembled twenty or thirty chairs (hey, we were optimistic), and then we waited. Eleven o'clock came and went, and no one showed up. Five more minutes passed. Still no one. We began to panic.

"Did we forget to put directions in the lobby?" Tina asked.

"I don't know. Maybe they're lost."

We looked at each other glumly, both thinking, but not saying, *Maybe they're just not coming.*

Suddenly the door opened and in walked our first guest, a woman named Mary Ellen Kullman, the new program director for the Arthritis Foundation. She was a delight, and her presence was immensely encouraging. Obviously the Arthritis Foundation believed in what we were attempting to do. There was just one problem: three people were now standing in the room, and I was the only one with arthritis! If this hadn't seemed so funny, we might have cried. As it was, we were laughing about "the world's smallest arthritis support group" when the door opened and a woman in her early thirties walked into the room. She was followed closely by a second young woman. I looked at Tina; Tina looked at Mary Ellen. Collectively, we let out a sigh of relief. Our membership had now nearly doubled!

Their names were Terri and Diane, and if they were at first nervous and self-conscious, they soon warmed to the setting. As the program founder, it was only fitting that I be the first to stand and bare my soul. I talked about my ninety-three days in the hospital and how I had come to the realization that helping myself meant more than just taking a lot of pills and seeing a lot of doctors; it meant understanding the adversary I was facing and trying to figure out how to deal with it on an emotional, physical, and spiritual level so that I could make better decisions and lead a better, more productive life. A big part of that, I explained, was meeting other people who had arthritis and being able to talk about the disease, sharing experiences about what works, and hopefully gain some wisdom in the process.

When I was finished, Terri and Diane related their stories. Each of them began by saying, in effect, "I can't believe I'm here. Do you know how excited I was to see your ad in the *L.A. Times*? A support group for young people with arthritis? Are you kidding me? I thought I was the only person in the world under fifty with this disease."

Like me, Terri had tried other support groups and found them well-meaning but not relevant to her situation. She felt isolated, adrift. "Not my husband, not my parents, not my employer. No one really understands. My boss thinks I'm either faking or nuts, and I don't blame him. One day I'm fine, the next day I'm too sick to work. Then I'm back the next day, and then I'm sick again. For someone who doesn't have arthritis, that's pretty hard to comprehend, isn't it?"

We all nodded our heads in agreement. The bonding was instantaneous. Our stories were different, yet powerfully linked by arthritis. Terri had driven more than an hour, from the South Bay area of Los Angeles, to attend this meeting; Diane, who lived in Pasadena, had driven even farther. It was no small inconvenience for each of us to get to this room, and yet we each had realized the importance of being there, of seizing this opportunity.

The conversation flowed freely, and so too did the tears. We'd tell horrific stories punctuated by moments of dark humor, and we were elevated by the discoveries of personal solutions. For more than two hours we laughed and cried, overwhelmed by the realization that we were no longer alone.

Yes! Yes! I feel the same way. I'm not crazy. It's not just in my mind!

It didn't take long to come to the conclusion that this group could be of enormous benefit. The verbal exercise of recounting our stories, even though parts of them were painfully sad, provided a catharsis that we had never experienced. This was an audience none of us had ever faced, an audience of our peers! Even our doctors, who were in the belly of arthritis on a daily basis, had no clue what it was really like twenty-four hours a day, seven days a week. They knew the proper descriptions and clinical terms, but they didn't have firsthand knowledge. They didn't know what it was like to hear your husband say, "What do you mean you can't have sex tonight? Why not?" They didn't know what it was like to hear your boss say, skeptically, "Came on you kind of suddenly, didn't it?"

Even Tina, who worked with arthritis patients every day, found the meeting to be an enlightening experience. She had never known that the pain and suffering could be so pronounced in a young person. "You know, when I think about it affecting me at my own age," she said after hearing the stories, "I get really scared. And I can understand now where you're coming from. I'm so accustomed to working with people who are sixty, seventy, eighty years old that I've never thought about how different the issues are for young people with arthritis."

The energy in that room, the heat generated by five people, felt like a revival! As facilitator, it was my responsibility to direct that energy, and so, in closing the meeting, I suggested that this was merely the first step of a new and beautiful journey. "I see us taking this to the next level. How many of you would like to have regularly scheduled meetings?"

Five hands shot up. My breath caught. I could barely speak. Young et Heart was about to take flight.

o   o   o

The brilliant anthropologist Margaret Mead once said, "Never underestimate the value of a group of committed volunteers," and she was so right. It dates back, in this country, anyway, to Revolutionary times, to the birth of the United States and the commitment of a group of passionate volunteers. It's the way almost anything of any value begins. Tina and I had no grandiose plans for Young et Heart. It had been born out of a very personal need: I wanted to connect with other young people. That's it. Nothing more. I needed help, the voice of experience, and didn't know where else to find it. But until I had met these other young women, I didn't know just how much I could learn. Suddenly Young et Heart seemed like not just a good idea, but a *cause*. The more people we could draw to our gatherings, the better.

So we decided to have another meeting in two months; after that, we would meet monthly. We agreed to bring in a speaker for our next meeting, someone who would address what we felt was the most important element of the disease: the psychosocial aspect of arthritis. In keeping with this theme, the meeting was titled "Getting Your Head Together About Arthritis." This time thirty-five people attended the meeting. To say we were thrilled would be a colossal understatement. We ran out of cookies, we ran out of coffee, we had to borrow chairs from another room. During the first hour of the meeting we went around the room and asked each person to introduce himself and summarize his story—what type of arthritis he had, how long he'd had it, and whatever else he wanted to share. The result was powerful. As we toured the room, one by one, people stood up, stated their names, told a bit of their stories, and broke down in tears.

"I can't believe I'm in a room with people just like me," one woman exclaimed.

"I've never met another young person with arthritis," said another.

"I can't even talk about this with my family," said one young man. "They think I'm crazy."

And so it went, for more than two hours. We shared our misery, and in so doing, the misery lifted—or at least, the weight of it seemed more manageable. For me, Young et Heart was a source of great pleasure, even as it exhausted me. What I would say to anyone with arthritis is this: Seek out others who share your pain, but more than that, try to alleviate their pain. Chronic illness often leads to depression, and when you're depressed you spend a lot of time thinking about yourself. You get so mired in your own suffering that you become disconnected from the rest of the world. Your discomfort becomes the center of your universe. But the more time I spent on Young et Heart, the more deeply I immersed myself in it, the stronger I became. My depression lifted, and I'm sure it was because I had a goal, and that goal involved helping other people.

The third meeting of Young et Heart attracted sixty people to Daniel Freeman Hospital. We were bursting at the seams! Again, we ran out of refreshments and chairs. People stood in the back of the room. It was an exciting, catch-the-fever type of atmosphere. When you're in a room with five people nodding their heads as you relate your story, it's a great feeling, but when sixty people are nodding . . . well, it's just inspiring. As before, a lot of people cried, but the feeling that permeated the room was not sadness, for these were tears of truth, of honesty, of brotherhood and sisterhood. Tears of hope.

Within three years the ranks of Young et Heart had swollen to nearly one thousand participants, with six different chapters, sponsored by six different hospitals and six different branches of the Arthritis Foundation, in the greater Los Angeles area. It grew like wildfire, fueled in no small part by a story that appeared in the *Los Angeles Times*. A reporter called me out of the blue one day and said,

"Hi, we understand you've put together something unique and we'd like to talk to you."

"On the phone? Now?" I scrambled for my notes and files.

"No, no, no. We'd like to send someone out to your house. Is that okay?"

"Sure, that would be fine."

I was living in Rolling Hills then, and deep into the surgical management program that would help make me whole again. At the time, however, I was surrounded by arthritis paraphernalia: wheelchairs, crutches, canes, etc. Sometimes I needed them, sometimes I didn't, but they were always around. The reporter seemed genuinely interested in both arthritis and Young et Heart.

"You're a dynamo," she said. "I don't know that I could have gone through something like this at your age. I don't think I would have handled it as well as you're handling it."

I laughed. "Quite frankly, for a long time I wasn't handling it very well at all. What you're seeing now is a butterfly. I used to be a caterpillar hiding in a cocoon, and this organization has helped transform me. I have a new kind of family now . . . a family of young people with arthritis . . . and the Arthritis Foundation."

The article appeared while I was at Daniel Freeman having another arthritis surgical procedure. I didn't know when it was going to be published, and found out in the oddest way. I received my morning newspaper as I always did, from a nice, elderly gentleman volunteer who made his rounds at the hospital each morning, always referring to me as "my girlfriend." At nine A.M. the phone system at the hospital opened up, allowing calls from the outside. At 9:02, the phone rang in my room. It was my mother . . . frantic.

"Have you seen that picture?!"

"*Uhhhh* . . . hi, Mom. How are you?"

"The picture, Amye. Have you seen the picture?"

"Mom, I don't have any idea what you're talking about."

She sighed, exasperated. "The article in the *Times* is out. Didn't you know?"

I looked at the paper, still folded in half at the foot of my bed. "What section?"

"Lifestyle," she said. "You're on the cover!"

I opened the paper, tossed aside the first two sections, and there I was, all over the cover of the *L.A. Times* Lifestyle section. I very quickly realized that my mother was not excited about the story; she was furious about the picture. And I understood why. It was terrible! On the day the photographer from the *Times* visited, I was wearing ratty blue jeans. He had asked me to lift my arms to give the reader an idea of what sort of reach I had, in spite of my arthritis. The resulting photo was a full-body shot of me doing some kind of Mae West thing—my arm propped up, my hand sort of pushing against my hair, as though I'm saying, *"Is that a crutch or are you just happy to see me?"* It was humiliating! The story didn't exactly thrill me, either. Beneath the painfully prosaic headline ARTHRITIS VICTIM FIGHTS PAIN WITH OPTIMISM was a treacly story laced with errors.

This whole experience taught me something about being careful when dealing with the media; it also taught me about the awesome power of the press, for despite its mistakes, the story had a galvanizing impact on Young et Heart. When I got out of the hospital, I returned to find that the tape on my home answering machine had run out. The *L.A. Times*, it seemed, had received a rash of calls following the publication of the Young et Heart story from young people wanting more information. The paper's response was to give out a telephone number, which they assumed was an office, but in fact was my home phone number. The reporter knew that I was willing to counsel people, but I certainly didn't expect my home phone number to be dangled as a prize. Then again, I didn't have a business number. I didn't even have a business! We had no organization, no office . . . *nothing*. Young et Heart was a group of volunteers trying to bring people together. So, even though I was upset about the way the newspaper handled the calls (they should have been referred to the Arthritis Foundation, of course), I was simultaneously invigorated by what they represented. So I rewound the tape and hit play.

"Hi! I read the story, and your group sounds great. I'd love to talk with you. How do I get in touch?" *Beep!*

"Hi . . . saw the article. Where are the meetings? I think they're at Daniel Freeman, but it didn't say exactly when and where." *Beep!*

"Hello, Ms. Leong. I work for a company that sells hot pads, and we'd like to chat with you about representation." *Beep!*

I spent a good portion of the next two weeks returning each and every one of those calls. If it was an inconvenience, it was a minor one, for it was a sure sign that Young et Heart was vital and needed. We built a network of young-adult groups around the country and in 1986 held our first half-day conference, entitled Arthritis in Prime Time, in Los Angeles. One hundred twenty-five people attended that first conference; within two years it had nearly quadrupled in size. Among the highlights of the 1988 conference, at the Los Angeles Hilton, was a fashion show for and about people with arthritis. Self-image is a major problem for most people with severe arthritis, but especially for young people. Your hands may be gnarled and withered, you don't walk quite like others, you have trouble standing, your clothes never seem to fit. As a result, you don't feel good about yourself or the way you look.

One of the things we wanted to show at this conference was that despite having arthritis, you can be happy with your appearance. (Beauty, after all, springs from within.) We wanted to help people figure out how to put on the appropriate makeup and choose the right clothes. For example, how do you zip up a dress when your shoulders don't work very well and you have no one to help you? I'd been on prednisone for a while and was extremely self-conscious about what it did to my face. From the neck down I looked like Twiggy, but my face was bloated and round, like a chipmunk's. I wanted to know how I could do my hair and makeup in such a way that my face wouldn't look so swollen. So I made a few calls and eventually was put in contact with a woman through Children's Hospital of Los Angeles named Sarah Richman, an aesthetician who had done some miraculous work with young burn victims. Sarah was a saint, as far as I was concerned. She utilized her magnificent skills to help children who had been viciously scarred, children who had already experienced a lifetime of pain and were now being subjected to the cruel taunts and stares of their classmates. Sarah, like so many others, was surprised to learn that young people got arthritis, but she needed little prodding to get involved in our project.

"Of course, I'd love to help," she said. We met for lunch and became instant friends. To this day, we affectionately call each other "sistah."

Sarah did a makeover session for women that proved to be one of the highlights of the conference, but perhaps the biggest success was our fashion show. In the months leading up to the conference we identified twelve young men and women with various types of arthritis, and we invited them to be models in our fashion show. At first, all of them declined.

"Are you crazy?!" one of them said. "I look awful."

"I don't need that kind of embarrassment," said another.

I kept after them, pleaded with them, assured them that we would do nothing to humiliate them or cause them any pain. And in the end they all agreed to take part. At the dress rehearsal, one week before the conference, our models were uniformly shy. They trudged, heads down, across the stage, like reluctant little kids. Nervous and apprehensive, they kept saying things like "Please, don't make me do this. Don't make me expose myself to all these people."

"Trust me," I said. "It'll be all right."

Sure enough, on the day of the fashion show, when they emerged from the dressing rooms with their brand-new outfits and their beautiful complexions and hairstyles (thanks to Sarah!), and they heard the applause of four hundred fifty people in the audience, they were reborn. As each model strutted proudly down the runway and across the stage, the audience heard about not just the clothes but the person beneath the clothes.

"This is Kathy," the emcee announced. "She's had rheumatoid arthritis for the past fourteen years, and she loves to read and garden."

Kathy just beamed. They all did, every one of our models. The transformation in just one week was nothing short of remarkable, and it reinforced my belief that we were on the right track. It was because of arthritis that we came together—for comfort, support, and education. But once we established a sense of community and trust and began to share our lives with others facing similar challenges, we discovered that we were so much more than our arthritis. Through friendship and a sense of purpose, we were transformed by one another. We became empowered by our own peers.

As I began to become more involved with the Arthritis Foundation as a volunteer, first at the local Southern California chapter level, then through the years at the national level, I met people who were to change my life for the better. Great and soulful people who just happen to have pretty bad arthritis like me. Linda Wilson of Massachusetts, Julia McClanahan from Tennessee, Janet Austin from Alabama, Norine Walker from Maryland, and Edie Nixon from Kentucky—all are dynamic, funny young characters who instantly became my "arthritis soul sistahs." We gave each other nicknames like Grits and Eggs, Dolly, and Cappuccino. Laughing through late-night all-girl pajama parties became part of our routine when we participated in national leadership meetings of the Arthritis Foundation. By day we were directing national policies and programs to help others with arthritis, and by night we were laughing and forming deep friendships of spirit, camaraderie, and soul. Because of arthritis, we had found in each other a depth of sisterly love and a passion for arthritis advocacy. Through our association as national volunteers of the Arthritis Foundation, we had formed a new family.

When I was elected chairwoman of the American Juvenile Arthritis Organization, a division of the Arthritis Foundation, we "soul sistahs" worked on projects targeted to help families, children, and young adults affected by childhood arthritis. One project involved vigorously educating Congress about the impact of arthritis on children and their families, and urging the declaration of a National Juvenile Arthritis Awareness Week. In 1990, after months of working with families and legislators across the country, Congress passed the declaration and noted that this movement achieved the rare accomplishment of touching families from every state in the union. Today, this campaign is continued by the Arthritis Foundation and educates more than 500,000 school kids and adults about the impact and need for early treatment of arthritis and the prevention of disability in young people. Our family of "sistahs" and new and old friends united on projects one after another for a common cause. The Arthritis Foundation became our oil and glue: as oil, it facilitated our capacity to speak out to government, the corporate world, and the medical community about the impact of arthritis on our young lives; and it provided us with the organizational glue to move our ideas into strategic actions with results. We saw and experienced the power of moving beyond our own pain to make positive changes in the way society viewed us. Powerful effect. Powerful medicine. Powerful relief.

Getting Close

One of the milestones of my arthritis journey occurred in my own room, while standing in front of a mirror. This was shortly before I was admitted to Daniel Freeman Hospital, when my weight had plummeted to seventy-nine pounds. I know there are some women who believe it isn't possible to be too thin, who are forever seeing fat where there is only bone, and who would view the image I saw this day as some sort of weird triumph.

Not me. I saw a corpse.

While cruelly assessing my naked body, as we women are wont to do on occasion, I was shocked by my own reflection. Swollen eyes and puffy, moonlike face sat on top of a stick. Sharp points jutted at odd angles from my hips, shoulders and knees; pale skin hung loosely from my frame. I ran a hand slowly across my rib cage, touched the bones protruding, counted them one by one, and felt a sickness rising in my throat. Who was this woman standing before me, and how had she reached such a sad, pathetic state? For the first time in my life, I seriously contemplated suicide. Not for long, mind you, but I did think about it. I thought, perhaps, that I'd be better off dead.

Who would miss me?

Who would really care?

The answer, of course, was my parents, my family, my friends. But, like most women, I wanted more than that. I wanted intimacy in my life. I wanted to love and be loved. And when I looked in the mirror and saw this ghastly . . . *thing* . . . staring back at me, I had to wonder: *Who would ever love me?*

Relationships, sex, self-image—these are baffling issues for those of us who bear the scars of arthritis. Pain and deformities have an interesting way of negating your sexual needs and desires. Other people's looks, stares, and subtle comments chip away at your confidence. You spend all your time trying to hide your illness—hide the way you walk, the way your arms and legs look, the way you feel. This is an emotionally painful and soul-deadening transformation, especially if you come from a place of confidence and comfort with regard to your own appearance. In high school, before I was diagnosed, I had been fortunate to be named homecoming queen and Christmas Formal queen. I worked for a time as a model in my hometown. People in our community encouraged me to enter the Miss Chinatown USA competition. I felt pretty good about my body and my self-image, and I understood the connection between looking good and feeling good. In the years after I was diagnosed with arthritis, I lost my confidence, my sense of self. It didn't happen overnight. Just as arthritis gnawed at my joints, it also took its toll by eating away at my self-image and how I projected myself to the opposite sex. I no longer felt like a woman.

I'd had a boyfriend or two before my diagnosis and in the early stages of the disease. While I was in college, I was fortunate to meet a new friend, a man named Adrien, who had returned to college after traveling and working at various jobs. He was a mature, sensitive man, and he became my first love. He was the first man with whom I developed a sensual relationship. I learned then, and am more certain now, that sensuality is the key to a complete and loving relationship. It isn't just about the sex act: jumping into bed. It's all about getting to know each other and learning to trust each other. But sensuality begins with the individual. It doesn't seep from the outside in, but rather exudes from the inside out. Your sense of self-confidence begins to emerge when you begin to care more about how you think and feel about yourself, and less about what strangers think of you. Confidence serves as a foundation from which to project your physical self to others. Sensuality is a natural by-product of feeling good about yourself—it practically flows through your pores for the world to see. Today, I understand this, but in the early days of my arthritis, sensuality and sexuality were just words.

My own ethnic heritage compounded the problem for me. Asian culture frowns upon demonstrative displays of sexuality. It also disapproves of displays of weakness or imperfection, and arthritis reflected both. Those two things, taken together, prompted me to shut down both emotionally and sexually. Adrien helped me break through this wall that I had built, largely because we established a strong bond of trust and friendship by spending time together, talking, laughing, and getting to know each other. This was a man who taught me that even though I had arthritis, and even though I hurt most of the time, it was okay to be with each other . . . to touch and explore each other. The sensuality of learning to communicate with my partner without words and without judgment or fear of rejection reconnected me to my feminine side. Like so many young women, I had been led to believe that sex was a tool, a way to convince a guy to fall in love with you. Arthritis made me question whether I had lost the use of that tool. But Adrien helped me question everything I had been taught. With him I could close my eyes and forget about arthritis, forget about what my ancestors were trying to tell me, and what they would say if they could see me.

As so often happens with first love, however, ours didn't last. We had different goals, different aspirations, and so we parted amicably. I had no way of knowing that it would be a very long time before I would find someone else who was capable of looking beneath the surface. With my days and nights consumed by arthritis, I had to set basic priorities, and my top priority was school. As it became increasingly difficult merely to get through each day, I devoted less and less time to matters of the heart. Subconsciously, too, I know that I was trying to hide. Arthritis had become a major part of my life, and yet, the stronger its grip, the harder I tried to pretend it didn't exist. I'd wear baggy pants, baggy shirts. I'd sit in the back row of the classroom. I expended vast amounts of energy trying to hide my affliction. Looking back, I can see now that my actions were motivated primarily by a loss of self-esteem.

Today, thankfully, I know that how you look is merely one small part of the equation. Personality, self-confidence, and character are equally important. When you walk into a room, people will give you the once-over, a two-second, up-and-down glance, but that's only the beginning. They'll also look at your eyes, the way you smile or don't smile, the way you interact with other people. Over the years, in metamorphosing from a caterpillar into a butterfly, I've learned to place a lot of emphasis on self-confidence.

I started out by sticking little affirmations on my mirror for me to see and say out loud each time I walked by. That may sound corny, but you'd be surprised at how effective it can be. (Research on depression management supports this notion of improving your attitude by verbally stating where you want to go.) Affirmations like "I'm beautiful inside and out" and "I have so much to offer this world" and "Every day in every way, I'm getting better and better" were taped to the mirror, silly as that might seem, and served as daily reminders that I was more than the sum of my malfunctioning parts. A few friends, after visiting my apartment, picked up on this. If they noticed I was sad or depressed, they'd say, "Amye, you have so much to offer. Don't let this ruin your life." Sometimes their words fell on deaf ears, but most of the time they didn't. It's amazing what a simple compliment can do for someone's self-esteem. I had been beating myself down so much that I just expected it from those around me. But when the most innocuous compliment would come my way, especially from friends who really knew me, I'd cherish the feelings it spurred.

Putting yourself together in a way that attracts another person is part of the male-female dance. But it's not purely physical. The ability to create conversation is equally important. For someone with severe arthritis, this may present a problem. How do you create interesting conversation when all you can think about is how bad you feel and how bad you look? For me, part of the answer was to become ridiculously well versed in current events and popular culture. I could talk about music, politics, sports, movies, books—almost anything—and this gave me an opportunity to demonstrate quickly to others that there was more to Amye Leong than what met the eye.

Today, when I conduct seminars, especially young-adult symposia, I'm often asked, "How do I talk about my arthritis? When do I bring it up?" Fair questions, because you never know what the reaction will be. I've met people over the years who believe that arthritis is contagious. Seriously! That shows you the ignorance faced by people who must cope with this disease on a daily basis. If you're in a dating situation and you'd like to share with your partner another layer of who you are, you may want to tell him or her about your arthritis. But "how" you proceed is key. The act of revealing something so personal, so important, might bring you closer.

Or not. There are no guarantees. I've had some horrific dating experiences because of my arthritis. On one date, after a few drinks and a nice meal, the conversation flowed easily. It wasn't until well into the date, when I excused myself to use the bathroom, that problems arose. We'd been seated at our table for nearly two hours, long enough for my joints to stiffen considerably. When I stood to walk to the bathroom, I moved slowly, awkwardly, like a robot. On the way back, while limping through the restaurant, I noticed my date staring at me. Realizing I had caught him, he quickly averted his glance. When I sat down at the table, it was as though I was suddenly sitting next to a different man. He didn't inquire about my condition, didn't ask why I was limping. In fact, he pretty much just stopped talking altogether. He was gone. Of course, I was partially responsible for that result. Today, I understand that being proactive and acknowledging stares with a short explanation might have saved the rest of that evening: *Yes, John, I do walk with a bit of a limp, especially when I've been sitting for a while. I have something called rheumatoid arthritis that's under control now with medications, but every now and then it let's me know when I've been sitting or standing too long.*

Years passed before I had the confidence to embrace this attitude, but slowly the wall around me began to crumble. I began to reclaim my passion for life and relationships.

Shortly after I had moved back to the Los Angeles area after being a ward of Mom and Dad for so long, I received an invitation to a neighborhood party. I had no intention of attending. I was just getting settled in my new home, I was still hobbling around on crutches, and although my attitude had improved tremendously, I wasn't yet prepared to hit the party scene. One night, though, while my friend Carol was visiting, she spotted the invitation.

"What's this?" she asked, fingering the card curiously.

"Oh, nothing. Just an invitation to a party in the neighborhood."

Carol looked at it more closely. She smiled. "Hey, it's a country-and-western party! I think we ought to go!"

With a frown, I dismissed the suggestion out of hand. "You can go. I'm not going anywhere. In case you hadn't noticed, Carol, I'm still on crutches."

"Oh, come on, Amye," she said. "You need to get out and meet some new people. There's no reason for you to be housebound."

"Sure there is. I can barely walk! And I look awful!"

Carol shook her head. "You look fine. And if you don't believe me, then maybe it's time to get another opinion." She tapped the invitation with her index finger. "This would be a good place to start."

"You don't give up, do you?"

"Uh-uh."

She didn't either. For the next three weeks, Carol worked on me. She teased, cajoled, flattered, shamed, and generally browbeat me into submission. In the end she talked me into going, and she did so by suggesting that I leave my crutches at home for the evening.

"Great idea," I said sarcastically. "Why not just cut off my legs while we're at it?"

"No, no, no. That's not what I mean. I'm going to be your crutches for the night. As soon as we leave this house, I'm your guardian angel; I'll watch over you, get you anything you need. If you have to use the bathroom, give me a signal, raise your hand, wink, whatever. If you want a new drink, just jiggle your glass."

"I don't know . . ."

"Trust me. It'll work. You just lean on me, sister."

When I finally relented, Carol went to work. She walked into my closet and began putting together a country-and-western outfit for me, one that would meet the strict criteria I had established.

"I know you're worried about people seeing your knees," she said, "So how about this?" She pulled out a long, denim skirt.

"Okay, I guess."

"Good." She returned to the closet, came out with a blouse, shoes, accessories—all in keeping with the country-and-western theme, and perfect for covering up the obvious signs of rheumatoid arthritis. Watching Carol work so hard at convincing me to have fun, I felt my reluctance melting.

"You know," I said, "this just might be okay."

Carol walked over and gave me a hug. "Of course it will. Like it or not, Amye Leong, it's time to start having fun again."

Carol drove to the party and double-parked in front of the house. As promised, my crutches were left behind. Now, at this time I had already had two surgical procedures on my feet, as well as one knee replacement. My surgical management program was under way, but I was still in pretty rough shape. Merely getting from the curb to the house, without assistance, would have been virtually impossible. But I had assistance. I had Carol. She helped me out of the car, gave me an elbow for support, and said, "Let's go."

We began walking very slowly, arm in arm, taking one small step, pausing to rest and recover, and then taking another small step. It took forever to get to the front door, and as other guests arrived they stopped and stared, doubtless wondering, *Who are these two strange women, and why are they walking in slow motion?*

Once inside the front door we continued our slow, steady march, arm in arm, Carol looking ahead, me looking at the floor, to make sure I didn't trip. I was extremely nervous about falling—that would have created a scene of unimaginable embarrassment. I envisioned myself crashing to the ground, pulling Carol along for the ride, screaming, crying, and then thrashing about on the floor like a fish out of water.

"Look up," Carol muttered under her breath. "Look up and smile, sweetie!"

"Get me to a chair," I said under my breath. "Then I'll smile."

After what seemed like an eternity, Carol finally got me seated safely on a couch, and immediately excused herself. "Gotta park the car. Be right back."

So, there I was, all alone, vaguely familiar with a handful of the guests, but friends with none of them. Within a few minutes, though, a man walked over, introduced himself as "William," and sat down next to me. We started talking, and as we talked, I began to laugh, quietly at first, but then more confidently.

"Everything all right?" he asked. It was a fair question, since he really hadn't said anything all that funny.

"Oh yeah, just fine."

The truth was, this man had me cornered. He could have been the homeliest man in the world (which he wasn't), had garbage breath (he didn't), and a repugnant personality (he was actually quite pleasant), and I still would have been a captive audience. He had my complete and undivided attention, because I literally could not move. And he didn't even know it. This struck me as downright hilarious.

When Carol returned, of course, she saw us together on the couch—William talking a mile a minute, me giggling like a school-girl—and immediately got the wrong idea.

"Well, looks like you're not having any problems," Carol said. "I'm going to wander for a while."

"Hey!" I protested, but she was gone.

I spent the next few hours on that couch, talking not only with this very nice gentleman but also with an assortment of other guests who stopped by to introduce themselves. As far I could tell, no one thought it was strange that I never moved from that spot. More likely, they just didn't notice. Everyone was still having a good time as the party came to a close and several of the guests suggested we meet at a nearby restaurant for a nightcap and a snack. In order to make a quiet departure, Carol and I let everyone else leave ahead of us. After nearly three hours, I was basically glued to that sofa; I could barely move at all. Carol helped me stretch, get the blood flowing, and after ten minutes or so, she finally hoisted me off the seat and into a standing position. What we didn't realize was that the owner of the house had been watching this entire procedure with a mixture of awe and concern. Sitting there all night, I must have looked like every other guest. But not anymore.

"Are you all right?" she asked.

"Yeah, it's no problem," I assured her. "Just my arthritis acting up. Takes me a little while to get moving if I've been in one position too long."

She nodded sympathetically. "Well, if there's anything I can do to help, just let me know."

Carol took her time with me, led me to the car patiently and gently, and gave me a pat on the back for being such a good sport. I had to admit that it had been an enjoyable evening, so much so that we decided to extend it a bit longer. Decked out in our cowgirl outfits, we drove to the restaurant and sauntered in arm in arm to meet the rest of the revelers. No sooner had we sat down than Carol noticed a striking gentleman looking our way. Wearing a sport coat, jeans, and cowboy boots, and with a neatly trimmed gray beard and thick silver hair, he bore a striking resemblance to country singer Kenny Rogers.

"I think he's looking at you," Carol said.

I laughed. "Yeah, right."

In a matter of seconds he was standing next to my chair, leaning down close enough for us to talk without having to shout over the music.

"Hi," he said warmly. "My name's Bob. I just had to come over and meet you."

"Oh?" I said, recognizing a line when I heard one, but not minding in the least—it had, after all, been awhile since I had played this game. "Why is that?"

He smiled. "Well, I've never met a Chinese cowgirl before."

I chuckled. "Yeah, I guess this looks pretty silly, huh?"

He shook his head. "Not at all. I think it's kind of cute."

For a moment I felt myself actually blushing; this, too, was a nice feeling, and one I hadn't experienced in some time.

We spent more than two hours in that spot, talking easily and comfortably about a number of different things. As closing time drew near, Bob offered to walk me to my car, which led to a minor panic attack. *Oh, God! Now he'll see me limping and want nothing more to do with me.* Rather than face that possibility, I brushed his offer aside. "No, that's all right. I can make it on my own. Why don't we just exchange phone numbers and we can talk again in a few days?"

He leaned in closer. "I am not leaving here until you let me escort you to your car. Please."

I sighed. *What have I got to lose? Might as well find out right now if this man is worth my time.* I proceeded to slide gingerly off the bar stool, but having sat for a long time, the stiffness made it nearly impossible to move smoothly. I grimaced as my feet hit the floor and my ankles absorbed my weight.

"Are you okay?" Bob asked. He had a look of horror on his face.

"Yeah," I said. "Just a touch of arthritis.

Bob nodded knowingly. "That can be pretty bad," he said, the tone in his voice reflecting sincerity and understanding. "I own horses. They have all kinds of problems with arthritis. It's very common."

"Really?"

"Uh-huh. And it hurts like hell, too."

I smiled through the throbbing in my ankles. "You've got that right."

Bob offered me his elbow and helped me to the door and out into the parking lot, all the while telling me about his horses and the laundry list of medications that had been prescribed for their arthritis, including cortisone and various anti-inflammatory drugs, most of which I, too, had taken at one time or another. It took us about ten minutes to cover the fifty-foot walk to my car—an effort hardly indicative of someone who had only "a touch of arthritis." It was more as if I had been zapped by a lightning bolt, and Bob knew it. He knew it, saw it with absolute clarity, and yet he didn't say a word. When we got to the car, Carol was waiting. Bob opened the door, helped me in, and said he'd give me a call.

"That would be nice," I said. And we drove off.

That evening represented the beginning of an eight-year relationship, during which my sense of sensuality and passion began to reemerge. Despite my fear of being rejected due to physical deformities, I found a gentle soul who saw beyond the crooked joints. His patience with me in sexual intimacy helped me to have patience with my physical limitations and my self-perception.

More recently, with a body full of at least a dozen surgical scars, my relationships have truly flowered. A handsome, intelligent gentleman named Evan has taught me how to see in myself the beauty of what I bring to him and the world. He doesn't see the scars or the deformed fingers or other physical limitations. He says he sees and is energized by the light in my eyes, the passion of my work, the brilliance of my smile, the kindness of how I treat him and others, and the sensual nature of our time together. I discovered, perhaps for the first time, that the sexiest part of a woman (and a man) is what's between your ears, not below your waist.

12

Passion and Opportunity

The success of our young-adult groups led to the opening of doors I had never even considered. In 1987, for example, I was invited to attend a national conference at UCLA conducted by C. Everett Koop, the United States surgeon general. Dr. Koop's office sponsored one or two major conferences each year focusing on important health topics. The focus of this particular conference was self-help and public health. Dr. Koop's staff had heard about my grassroots work with Young et Heart and had contacted me to discuss the program in greater detail. Several interviews followed, in which I not only told my story and the evolution of Young et Heart, but also provided my own definition of self-help and its value in bringing together people who face similar challenges. Apparently they liked my answers, because one day in the summer of 1987 I received a letter from Dr. Koop asking if I would like to be one of the two hundred people taking part in his conference on self-help. It took me all of three seconds to respond affirmatively.

What I didn't know at the time was that no one else from the arthritis community had received an invitation to take part in this conference. Given the fact that I was so new to the field, this was an amazing development, and one that might have both disturbed and overwhelmed me had I been aware of it at the time the invitation was extended. Arthritis, after all, affects tens of millions of people, and while my case was particularly brutal, I was hardly an expert. My career in advocacy wasn't really even a career yet—I was still living on disability and trying to juggle my responsibilities as a volunteer advocate with the Arthritis Foundation with my own surgical management program. Surely there were others more qualified than I to attend a conference headed by the most powerful and influential man in American health care.

Nevertheless, as the conference drew near my trepidation dissipated. Maybe there were bigger names in arthritis, physicians and scientists with resumes as long as their arms, but no one felt more strongly than I did about the importance of self-help and advocacy. If I was nervous, it was only because I was so excited about having an opportunity to meet others with a similar passion.

The conference was held in September. We spent three days formulating recommendations for the surgeon general on how we could assist self-help groups in our respective communities and across the country; how we could develop new partnerships involving potential support from the federal government; and what the government could do to promote this grassroots movement. The two hundred participants were divided randomly into groups on the first day of the conference. Each group had a facilitator (to guide discussions) and a recorder (to record the events of each meeting). At the end of the day, the facilitators and recorders would get together and evaluate the groups' progress. Although I was new to the process, I thought we worked hard and efficiently, and I was pleased with what we accomplished. Still, I was surprised on the last day when a conference leader walked into our room, approached our facilitator, and whispered into his ear. The facilitator then looked in my direction and said, "Amye, would you please step outside for a moment?" I felt like I'd been hurled back in time twenty years, to one of those terrible days in elementary school when you're summoned to the principal's office and you have no idea what you've done wrong.

Slowly I got up out of my chair. I was still relying on crutches at this time, but I had chosen not to use them at the conference because I didn't want to call attention to myself or deal with a litany of explanations. There were thirty-five people in the room and it felt as though they were all staring at me as I slowly hobbled through the doorway, sweat building on my brow with each halting step.

In the hallway was a woman I recognized from the opening ceremony of the conference. Her name was Fran, and she was smiling pleasantly as I approached. "Hi, Amye," she said, extending a hand. "We'd like to ask a favor of you."

"What is it?"

"Dr. Koop is going to be conducting a press conference this afternoon, shortly after the closing ceremony, and we'd like you to represent the participants from the conference."

My jaw dropped open. "You're kidding, right?"

She shook her head. "Uh-uh. We'd like you to sit at the front table, right next to Dr. Koop. The media will ask some questions, most directed at Dr. Koop, but some will probably be asked of you. They'll want to know your personal history, how you came to be at the conference, and what you thought of it—things like that. If you'd like to defer to Dr. Koop, then go right ahead."

She paused, smiled.

"Of course, he may defer to you at times, too."

"Oh, please."

"I'm serious," Fran said. "You're not merely window dressing here."

I asked why they had chosen me, I wasn't even a group leader.

"We wanted someone who could speak on behalf of the group from different perspectives," she explained, "but mostly from the perspective of someone intimately familiar with self-help; someone eloquent who is not only involved with self-help, but is a benefactor of the self-help process. That's you."

I accepted the offer and listened as Fran described what would happen. "We'll all convene as a group and make our recommendations. Then we'll close out the conference. Dr. Koop will walk out with his entourage of people, down the center of the aisle and out the back door. From there he'll go directly to the press conference. You'll join us every step of the way."

Every step of the way.

Interesting choice of words. I should have responded with, "Oh, by the way, I walk *really* slow." But I didn't. I just said, "I'd be honored," and left it at that.

So we went through the whole ceremony. Dr. Koop made his closing remarks, everyone applauded, and we began to file out, all of us proud of the work we had done and filled with a sense of accomplishment. Dr. Koop, wearing his crisp, white surgeon general's uniform, left the room trailed by a phalanx of some twenty community leaders. He very quickly passed me and just kept on walking, didn't even acknowledge me—but then, why would he? I was just one of two hundred people.

While waiting for everyone to pass, I stood and tried to work out the kinks in my joints. We'd been sitting for two hours, and I was pretty stiff by then. Then I hustled after Dr. Koop and his entourage, trying my best to catch up so that I wouldn't be late for the press conference. Unfortunately, by the time I got to the doors of the auditorium, Dr. Koop and his people were already down the steps and halfway across a plaza that separated the auditorium from the site of the press conference. They were perhaps fifty yards ahead of me. Suddenly, I started to panic.

Oh, my God! How am I going to get down all of these steps? The press conference will be over by the time I get there.

Not knowing what else to do, I yelled for help. "Hey! Wait for me!"

The man in white stopped on a dime (nearly causing a chain-reaction collision among the entourage), turned, and looked at me. He pointed at himself, as if to say, "Are you talking to me?"

"Yes!" I shouted.

Dr. Koop nodded and waved. The message was clear: *Come join us!*

I proceeded to limp gingerly down the steps, one at a time, very, very slowly. Everyone could see there was something wrong, so Dr. Koop broke away from the crowd and walked in my direction. By the time I got to the bottom of the steps, he was waiting for me.

"Hi, Dr. Koop. My name is Amye Leong, and I've been asked to join you at the press conference. I'm representing the conference participants."

"Very nice to meet you, Amye," he said. He gave me a quick up-and-down glance and added, "What do we have here anyway?"

"Rheumatoid arthritis. I've had a lot of surgery and I'm really doing much better now—I used to be in a wheelchair—but walking is still not one of my best activities."

With that, Dr. Koop held out his arm for me. "You just take as much time as you'd like." For the remainder of the walk, the pace of the group was my pace: slow and deliberate. And I remember thinking, *What a sweet and gentle man.*

The press conference was held at the UCLA Faculty Club. When we arrived, everyone was milling about. There were only two chairs in the holding area: Dr. Koop took one and offered the other to me. Everyone else stood. While waiting for the media to set up, Dr. Koop and I had a delightful conversation. We talked about the success of the conference and the initiatives that had grown out of it, and I sensed that he was legitimately concerned about the issue of self-help; he did not strike me as a typical bureaucrat. As the press conference began, a can of soda was placed in front of each of us. Dr. Koop immediately popped his open and took a drink—the lighting was intense, and we both were sweating. I wanted a drink, too; however, the condition of my hands was such that pulling the tab on a can of soda was a task of insurmountable difficulty. My throat was parched and I feared that I'd be unable to speak, so I pushed the can closer to Dr. Koop, who knew instinctively what to do. As he addressed the media he reached over, took the can of soda, quickly opened it up, and handed it back, all without missing a beat or interrupting a sentence. I was impressed. He had all the qualities of a great surgeon general: the combination of sensitivity, compassion, and dexterity.

A few months later, in January 1988, I received another call from Dr. Koop's office. It's funny, when you get a call from the surgeon general, it's as if the president were calling: you feel an overwhelming urge to stand up and salute while you're on the phone. You feel as though you need to brush your teeth, comb your hair, and put on something presentable. It's that intimidating.

I had enjoyed the self-help conference immensely and had found Dr. Koop to be a warm, sincere, intelligent, eloquent gentleman, so I was very excited to hear from anyone in his office. On the phone was a woman named Heddy Hubbard, one of Dr. Koop's assistants. She invited me to meet with Dr. Koop and his staff to discuss the various recommendations that had come out of the conference. I was thrilled! Here I was, just this petite young woman, half crippled, going through all these joint-replacement surgeries so that she could lead a productive life, and now I was being asked to work directly with the surgeon general of the United States. What an honor!

Within five weeks I was in Bethesda, Maryland, at the office of the surgeon general, helping his staff develop an organization that would serve as an advisory board in the area of self-help. Dr. Koop wanted to know how he could best use his substantial power and influence to move this concept along. Now, most of us, when we think of self-help, think of a small group of like-minded people getting together to share their experiences and knowledge. We think of groups like Alcoholics Anonymous, groups that begin at the grassroots level. Young et Heart was like this, too. For the very first time, though, under Dr. Koop's leadership, self-help came to have broader credibility. It became part of a series of actions led by a person who had the power within a governmental structure to say, "This is good for the health of Americans, and we're going to do this on a national level." In a society where so much money was being spent on health care, and yet the emotional and empowerment needs of people dealing with disease were not being met, having the concept of self-help embraced by Dr. Koop was a major coup. At its core was a burgeoning movement of volunteerism, of people getting fired up and taking matters into their own hands, and now the surgeon general was endorsing it, publicly acknowledging its value. That alone, to me, was enough. That he was also saying, "Okay, Amye, help us mold it, help us develop an organizational structure that will allow me to use my position as surgeon general to affect all the other government agencies that deal with health, so that we can begin to educate them on the value of self-help, and implement programs in American communities." Wow! What an opportunity. And what a responsibility.

I began making monthly trips across the country to work with the surgeon general's office, and a small group of self-help leaders. This was no small task given my ever-changing physical condition. On one of the trips I had skewers protruding from my toes because of another round of foot surgery. The bones were falling out of alignment and the joints were becoming loose, so they had to "redo" one of my earliest surgical procedures, although this time I opted to have both feet done at the same time.

For this particular trip I had already purchased an economy ticket (the government was picking up the tab, after all) from American Airlines, but I was going to somehow have to keep my feet elevated the entire flight to minimize pain and swelling. Try that in coach class! I spoke to a representative of American and he was very courteous and accommodating, and also quite concerned. When I arrived at the airport and they saw the little green-tipped metal rods sticking out of my toes, they quickly upgraded my ticket to first class. The flight attendants were wonderfully gracious and helpful. I advised them that if anyone bumped my feet I would have no choice but to scream, for the pain of even the slightest bump was excruciating. They listened, and the trip went smoothly.

Traveling with arthritis, or any other kind of mobility impairment, is challenging. On this particular flight it was pretty obvious that I had a serious problem—crutches and feet implanted with metal skewers are a dead giveaway—but on subsequent trips I discovered that the situation can be more complicated when the disability is less obvious, because you are literally on your own. You have to connect all the dots ahead of time: *I have to get from my home to the car, from my car to the shuttle, from the shuttle to the terminal, from the terminal to the jetway. I have to deal with my heavy luggage. I have to get situated in a position where I won't disturb anyone else by being unable to move out of the way. I may not be able to open a tray table or adjust my seat or reach the call or light button.* I trained myself in those days to be aware of everything, to walk through the entire journey in my mind well ahead of time and to plan accordingly for my needs. Even now, when I can move with a good degree of fluidity and normality, I still do that, and I strongly recommend it for anyone with mobility difficulties who has to travel. I'd also like to say to those of you who are fortunate to be able-bodied . . . *slow down.* I know we're all running around, leading hectic, even chaotic lives, but try to make room for sensitivity. I'm not talking about charity or pity. I'm talking about awareness. People walk slowly for a variety of reasons, but when you see someone having trouble opening a door or trying to pick something up, even though you're in a rush and the world is moving fast, try to have some respect and some compassion. Offer assistance whenever possible. Believe me, your kindness will be appreciated. For those of you who have arthritis and need some help, don't be shy about asking for it, because ultimately it is your responsibility.

Dr. Koop named seventeen people to his new advisory body, which was called the National Council on Self-Help and Public Health, an impressive group of people at the top of their respective fields. They represented the American Hospital Association, the American Medical Association, large self-help groups such as Alcoholics Anonymous, and cancer support groups. There were eminent psychologists, sociologists, internationally known writers and scholars, people from all walks of life who were interested in advancing self-help. We became a family team of Koop's advocate army. To my surprise and delight, Dr. Koop named me to this advisory board; to my utter amazement, at the very first meeting, I was elected chairwoman.

One of the great things about believing in a cause is that you don't have the luxury of intimidation. If these people respected me enough to chair their board, then I would do it, and I would throw myself into it heart and soul. We quickly developed an action plan, the first step of which was to meet with leaders of the government's Public Health Service. We educated them about self-help. We talked to them about the importance of using the strength of the federal government, of dangling grant money as a carrot. We encouraged them to incorporate self-help into their national and community-based programs. Hundreds of self-help and mutual-help groups began popping up all over the country, and we offered funding support for things like self-help clearinghouses and toll-free hot lines in different parts of the country that would provide information and direction to anyone who needed help with a particular affliction. If you called and related your disease or areas of interest, you'd be given contact numbers and resources. Today this is an expected component of health care, but it was a novel concept in the late 1980s.

Dr. Koop was supportive of our strategic efforts. Sadly, one of the things I learned is that dealing with the federal government is like dealing with the weather: when the wind shifts, everything changes. During the course of Dr. Koop's tenure, he became quite vocal about tobacco and the role of tobacco companies in consumer usage. He became vocal about abortion. And, of course, he was highly outspoken about HIV and AIDS. Inevitably, perhaps, given his increasing popularity, he fell out of favor with the Bush administration, and nearing the end of his term we received word that all of Dr. Koop's self-help initiatives would be ending. Just like that. But it was fun and inspiring while it lasted, and I've seen that the work we did lives on today. At the very least, it taught me the power of government, and the importance of getting involved, of fighting inertia and complacency. I didn't have a medical degree or a Ph.D. I was not the head of a Fortune 500 company. I was a person with a serious disability and a desire to help others similarly afflicted. All I had was firsthand, experiential knowledge of arthritis and a passion to help others, and yet somehow, almost as if by fate, that has led to a whole new life.

By 1991, advocacy and activism had become the center of my ever-expanding universe. I was traveling around the country, speaking to local chapters of the Arthritis Foundation, working with various health organizations, and finally scratching out a living. New and exciting opportunities seemed to present themselves almost monthly. One such opportunity came in the form of a phone call from Dr. Fred McDuffie, the former medical director of the Arthritis Foundation.

"Amye," he began, "I'm sitting here looking at a lovely picture of you and me and a few Japanese women. And in this photo, someone has taken a pen and drawn a circle around you."

"Really? Why is that?"

"Well, it's accompanied by a letter from the Japan Rheumatism Society," he said. Now it was coming back to me. A year or so earlier, during an anniversary celebration of the Arthritis Foundation, I had met a woman from the Japan Rheumatism Society. We were the only Asian women in the room and somehow we had gotten together and become friendly, even though I didn't speak a word of Japanese and she didn't speak a word of English.

"What does the letter say?" I asked.

Dr. McDuffie began to read. "I can't remember this young woman's name," the letter said, "but we met in your country last year, and we would like to invite her to Japan to speak at our anniversary event."

I was honored. "That's so sweet, Fred. Are you going, too?"

He chuckled into the phone. "Amye, they didn't invite me."

Oops!

"I'll forward the letter and you can respond," he said, letting me off the hook. "Personally, I think it's a great opportunity and I encourage you to go."

Actually, I didn't need much encouragement. I'd never been to Japan before, and I hoped to use this invitation as an opportunity to visit other Asian countries, including the land of my ancestors. My sister accompanied me on the trip, largely because it was going to be an exhausting, challenging adventure made doubly so by the fact that I was still using one crutch to get around.

The night before the formal anniversary conference, we attended a reception for some four hundred guests at an elegant Tokyo ballroom. There were three honored guests: a woman from the United Kingdom, a gentleman from Germany, and "Miss America," which was what they named me. After opening remarks and a discussion of the next day's agenda, the mistress of ceremonies led the entire group in a giant sing-along. Everyone in the room, with the notable exception of the "honored guests," knew the lyrics. Still, it was a beautiful experience, karaoke at its best. After the first song, they launched right into another. Finally, that song ended, and it seemed time to dig into the feast that awaited (I mean *feast!* Mountains of crab legs, lobster, sushi, giant prawns resting on boats of carved ice!). To my horror, however, the mistress of ceremonies walked to our table, leaned over, thrust a microphone in my face, and said, in heavily accented English, "Okay, you sing now!"

I panicked. I started looking for the closest exit, because if there's one thing I don't do, it's sing. Oh, maybe in the shower once in a while, or driving down the highway with the windows rolled up when my favorite tune comes on the radio. But in public? Not this bionic babe!

I shook my head vigorously, tried to push the microphone away, and said. "Oh, no. Really. I can't."

"You sing!"

"I'd rather not."

"You sing!"

The audience was applauding now and the mistress of ceremonies was tugging at my arm. So I stood up and, reflexively, grabbed the shoulder of the woman from the United Kingdom, who was seated next to me. "Come on, I'm not going up there alone."

"What?" she cried. And suddenly there we were, the two of us walking toward the stage.

"Think of a song—quick!" I implored her.

"How about . . . 'My Bonnie Lies over the Ocean'?"

" 'My Bonnie Lies over the Ocean'?"

"That's the best I can do."

I took a deep breath, closed my eyes, and started singing.

"My Bonnie lies over the ocean . . . My Bonnie lies over the sea . . ."

And so two people who had never before sung in a public setting got through a wretched version of "My Bonnie Lies over the Ocean." Bad as it was (and believe me, it was *very* bad), the audience applauded warmly. We had survived! As I started to nudge my counterpart from the UK off the stage, the mistress of ceremonies rushed at us again, smiling and clapping enthusiastically.

"No, no, no," she said. "You sing another song!"

She gestured to the audience, which burst into applause again. I looked at the woman from the UK. She shrugged her shoulders. "I'm out of songs. You come up with one this time."

It's odd how the mind works. I love music. There are hundreds of songs to which I know the lyrics, and yet at that moment my mind went completely blank. Instead of coming up with the name of some Beatles song I love, or a favorite ballad, all I could think of was "I've Been Working on the Railroad." I'm not kidding. Those are the words that came out of my mouth.

"Do you know that one?" I asked my new partner.

"I think so, but I'll have to follow your lead."

So, as if to perpetuate a Western stereotype, this Chinese-American warbled the chorus of "I've Been Working on the Railroad." The audience rose from their seats in applause. We were an American hit in Japan!

As we walked off the stage, a young Japanese woman on crutches stopped me and said, "I'd like to sing a song with you." By now I was beyond the point of embarrassment, so I asked her what she would like to sing.

She leaned forward and whispered into my ear, "Do you know the words to 'We Shall Overcome'?"

I didn't, but I followed her lead, and the two of us began to sing:

> We shall overcome . . .
> We shall overcome . . .
> We shall overcome . . . some . . . day!

We knew only the chorus, so we sang it twice, and when we finished the audience rose as one. They gave us a standing ovation! I turned to this young Japanese woman and, with tears welling in my eyes, embraced her as a sister.

This moment was about young people with arthritis around the world trying to overcome a disease that most people think only comes with age. We were the two youngest people in the room, and despite the differences in geography, culture, and language, we agreed that from that day forward, we would always be connected, like family, in our passion to make a difference for young people with arthritis. In just one evening, I was embraced by the love of Japanese arthritis advocates, and realized just how small the world really is. I would never feel alone again.

One of the reasons I wanted to visit Asia was to address my illness in terms of my heritage. I'd spent a good deal of my life being embarrassed by my arthritis, and I sensed at some level that this was attributable to the fact that I am of Asian ancestry. Self-esteem is linked to the culture in which you are raised. In my family there is still a very strong Asian perspective, and when I was growing up, I was taught that if you had a flaw, you didn't discuss it. You didn't show it. So I really began to feel a need to look at my illness not just as a woman, or as an American, but as a person of Chinese descent, and what I discovered was something truly remarkable.

The predominant reaction in Asia to illness in general, and arthritis in particular, is shame, and I found through my travels that nowhere is this more true than in mainland China. In Japan, people cast glances but, out of respect, said nothing when they saw me on my platform crutches. In Taiwan, where the motor scooter is among the most popular modes of transportation, and where crosswalks are merely a suggestion, people stared openly at me. They would whiz by on scooters, nearly knocking me off my crutches, and as they sped away they would turn around and stare, even point. It had been some time since I'd felt like I was part of a circus sideshow, but that feeling returned in Taiwan. None of that, however, was adequate preparation for mainland China. As one of the travel guides who led us from Hong Kong into China explained, "In China, people like you don't go out in public." When I heard that I was shocked, and insulted. Here I was, a woman of independent, entrepreneurial spirit, facing an attitude of my own ancestors that had total disregard for what I was all about as a human being.

In the end, though, it was an enlightening journey. When we visited a small village in southern China, an elderly woman came up to me as we were walking through the marketplace. This was a very small, impoverished town: no running water, outdoor rest rooms, that sort of thing. In the middle of the market, surrounded by hanging ducks and goat heads, this tiny woman grabbed one of my crutches and started yelling. She was shaking, crying. So I called to one of the guides and said, "What is she saying?" He listened for a moment, then pointed to my crutch and said, "She wants to know where she can get one of those." My heart sank. Obviously she was in pain and having trouble walking. I knew the signs of arthritis, and this poor old woman exhibited most of them. I let her try my crutches, which were too tall for her, and then explained, through an interpreter, that she would need to see her doctor to obtain a set of her own.

"See your doctor," I said again.

She gave me a hard look. *"Doc-tor?"* Then she shook her head, turned, and walked away.

It was such a poignant little moment, and I realized, there but for the grace of God go I. When I got back to the tour bus, I thought about this woman and the life she was leading, a life that would be even sadder, harder, because now she knew something was out there that could help her, something as simple a crutch, but something that she might never have, any more than she would have access to good-quality medical care.

"Doc-tor?"

I recalled her thin, frail voice, and I broke down and cried.

13

Torchbearer

There are moments in every life that are so wondrous, so unexpected that they steal your breath away. I remember
hobbling to the mailbox one cool morning in the winter of 1996,
anticipating nothing out of the ordinary, and being overwhelmed
by what I discovered. There, tossed in among the usual assortment
of postal debris—credit card solicitations, bills, shrieking sweep-
stakes come-ons—was a simple, but startling, one-page letter.

> *Dear Amye:*
>
> *Congratulations! You have been selected as a Community Hero
> Torchbearer for the 1996 Olympic Torch Relay. In honor of the out-
> standing contributions you have made to others in your community,
> I would like to personally invite you to carry the Olympic Flame, the
> most sacred symbol of the Olympic Movement.*
>
> *For 84 days, beginning April 27, the 1996 Olympic Torch Relay
> will bring the Olympic Flame to thousands of communities across*

America. You have been selected by a panel of community leaders from your region as one of the individuals who will represent the best of their community by carrying the Olympic Flame.

Please read the enclosed information carefully. It briefly explains the 1996 Olympic Torch Relay and the important role you will play as a Torchbearer. The final page is a Confirmation of Participation that must be completed and returned no later than February 5. Once you have confirmed your participation in the Torch Relay, we will forward more detailed information.

I hope you will accept this prestigious honor to participate in the Olympic Movement and carry the Olympic Flame. I look forward to your response and your involvement in the 1996 Olympic Torch Relay.

With best regards, I am

Sincerely,
William Porter Payne
President and CEO
The Atlanta Committee for the Olympic Games

At first I thought it was a hoax. I laughed out loud and started to crumple the letter, even before I had finished reading it. Then I fumbled through the attachments. On the last page, in bold print, was the name of the person who supposedly had nominated me for this honor: Bob! Over the course of the past two years, our relationship had ended but we had rekindled our friendship. Bob had come to understand my need for independence; I think he was even proud of what I had accomplished. Until that moment, though, I did not realize just how proud he must have been.

I rushed to the phone and began dialing Bob's number.

"You're kidding?" he said, when I told him about the letter. "You got it? I can't believe it! You really got it!"

His enthusiasm, of course, said a lot about our relationship. In a sense, it was deeper now than it had been when we were lovers, and I felt fortunate to call him my friend.

It wasn't long, however, before the excitement of being chosen to carry the torch was replaced by a serious case of anxiety. There is something wonderfully romantic about the Olympic torch and the spirit it represents. Every four years the Olympic flame travels from Athens, Greece, the site of the first Olympic Games, to the site of the upcoming Olympiad. The journey can be seen not only as a symbol of the enduring appeal of peaceful, athletic competition among nations but also as a metaphor for struggles great and small, and I was enthralled by the idea of participating in this ritual. Practically speaking, though, I was ill equipped for the venture.

While sharing the news with Bob—and, subsequently, my parents and a few other close friends—I kept envisioning myself jogging gracefully, elegantly through the streets of Los Angeles, the torch held aloft, its flame flickering against the sky high above my head. Then I remembered something: *Wait a minute . . . I can't run!* Well, that's not entirely true. I suppose if my life depended on it, I could hobble faster than usual. But I can't really *run*. I have artificial knees. I've got osteotomies in my toes. I've got plastic and metal parts everywhere. Even though I literally have been rebuilt from the ground up, I don't have strength. I don't have endurance. I'm doing the best I can with a fork and spoon right now. I'm happy that I can walk. I'm happy that on good days I don't need crutches. But running is not really an activity that's recommended for someone who has severe rheumatoid arthritis. The pounding on the pavement can seriously jeopardize the longevity of the prosthetic pieces. Naturally, it wasn't long before that image of a confident, athletic woman striding smoothly through the streets was replaced by the image of a pathetic woman stumbling and falling and setting her hair on fire.

I wanted to accept the invitation, but I was afraid of the consequences. I didn't want to embarrass myself; more important, I didn't want to be responsible for turning the Los Angeles leg of the Olympic Torch Relay into some sort of a circus sideshow. If it could be done safely, and with dignity, then I would happily, gratefully, take part. Otherwise, I would have to be satisfied with being a spectator.

Some of my concerns were allayed when I contacted the organizers of the event. First of all, I was not the only person with a disability who had been asked to carry the torch. All the community heroes were distinguished by characteristics or deeds that the committee deemed to be in some way "inspirational." Some of us were physically challenged; most were not. They were people who had performed some sort of heroic act. For, example, one of the community heroes was a fireman who had rescued a child from a burning building. There was a policeman, too. In my mind, these are the kinds of people who are truly heroic—people who make a decision to be courageous, to place their lives in jeopardy when they do not have to. I don't think of myself as being particularly heroic or courageous, because my condition was foisted upon me. I would never *choose* to have rheumatoid arthritis, or to have most of my major joints replaced. My only choice is in how I will deal with the obstacles the disease presents to me. Still, if others find my actions to be inspiring, well, that's wonderful. I'm flattered. So I was deeply honored to be part of this group.

Even more encouraging was the committee's response when I said, quite frankly, that I was not capable of running, nor could I lift a four-pound torch over my head.

"You know, I have rheumatoid arthritis," I told them.

"Yes."

"Well, I have artificial shoulders, artificial elbows, artificial fingers, reconstructed wrists. I can't lift two pounds, let alone four pounds. Incidentally, how tall is the torch and flame?"

"About forty-eight inches."

"Good lord! And you want me to keep it extended out in front of me, so that it's as far away from my head as possible?"

"Only makes sense, don't you think?"

"Uhhh . . . yeah. But how do I do that."

"That's up to you, Amye. Be as creative as you want to be."

The torch was scheduled to arrive in Los Angeles in late April and then spend the next three months snaking its way across the United States, eventually landing in Atlanta, Georgia, site of the 1996 Summer Olympics. In towns and cities all over the country it would be escorted by literally thousands of people—celebrities, athletes, politicians, and community heroes. My invitation had come in January, so I had three months in which to devise a plan that would allow me to successfully cover the meager six-tenths of a mile that constituted my leg of the relay. I started out by querying all my friends and relatives. Then I turned to the Internet. I went on line and asked for ideas. I explained my situation and my disability and said that I would welcome any help I could get. In short order I received about fifty responses, some silly, some clever. One person wrote: "Have four men carry you on a chair, over their heads, like an Egyptian princess." I liked that one. Less appealing was the suggestion that I be wrapped inside a rug and rolled along the torch route. There were all kinds of crazy, funny ideas, some of which I even passed along to the Olympic committee. Each time I was politely but firmly reminded of the event's guidelines, the most stringent of which was: "You must do it alone."

So I approached a company called Electric Mobility, which manufactures different types of scooters and motorized wheelchairs for people with varying degrees of mobility impairment. I said, "Look, I'm a spokesperson for the Arthritis Foundation, I have rheumatoid arthritis, I've initiated support groups all over the country, and I have just been asked to carry the Olympic torch as one of L.A.'s community heroes. Would you like to help me . . . *please!?*" And they jumped at the opportunity. They loaned me a wonderful little souped-up scooter that we painted red, white, and blue. I then had my means to travel six-tenths of a mile. I went back to the committee and said, "Is it okay if I use a scooter?" To which they replied, "Absolutely. As long as you're the only one on board."

The next step was to begin training. On the weekends I met my family in Fresno, and we worked together in an effort to whip me into shape. We started out by filling a big jug with enough water so that it weighed about four pounds. I was to practice holding it above my head while driving the scooter. Well, I couldn't lift it to my shoulders or even walk with it. My mother, sister, niece, little Amye, and nephews, Nick and Christopher, were sitting in the bleachers, watching me struggle, and they were shaking their heads, saying, "Nope, this isn't going to work."

It soon became obvious that even if I pumped a lot of iron, worked with a physical therapist and a personal trainer, there was no way that I could muster up enough strength to carry this thing. So we all agreed that we'd have to come up with another solution. Not only did I need a mode of transportation; I also needed a special holder for the torch.

That's when I decided to approach a friend, Dena Slonaker, who was the director of occupational therapy at HealthSouth, the largest rehabilitation company in the United States.

"Dena," I said. "I need your help. I've been invited to participate in the Olympic Torch Run. But, as you know, I have a little problem: I can't run and I can't carry a torch. Do you think your company would get behind me? I don't know if we'll be allowed to advertise, so I don't know what I can do for you in return, but I would love HealthSouth to be a part of this whole endeavor. What do you think?"

Dena wasted no time in responding. "Let me run it by my supervisors," she said. "But I think I can talk them into it."

Within a few days Dena called me back. She was very excited. HealthSouth was on board! So now I had two national companies supporting me in my effort to carry the Olympic torch. I couldn't believe my good fortune.

After talking with Dena and some of her staff, we decided that the only practical way to approach the project was to bring my scooter to the HealthSouth facility in Van Nuys, California, and let their occupational therapists work with it on-site. There they began the remarkable creative process of adapting the scooter into something that I could use in the torch run. Designing an ordinary torch holder was complicated enough; compounding the difficulty was an Olympic Committee stipulation that I needed to actually touch the torch in order to comply with the rules; the connection between the torchbearer's hand and the torch itself is a fundamental component of the philosophy of the relay. Therefore, somehow, I had to drive the scooter while grasping the torch. This was no small challenge— for me or the designers.

To my astonishment they were able to provide me with the means to conquer this problem by creating a torch holder that was molded to the arm of the scooter. It was a strange blue contraption adorned with lips and cups, as well as an elbow rest. The first time I saw it, I was awestruck by the sheer ingenuity that had gone into its design. Whether it would work was another matter.

Fortunately, the Olympic Committee was equally supportive. Two weeks before the event, they allowed me to take temporary possession of the torch so that we could complete the modification of the scooter and do a test run. Representatives of the Olympic Committee actually came out to Van Nuys, along with a television crew from the local NBC affiliate. A reporter had contacted me earlier and said, "We're querying some of the community heroes to find out what they're doing to prepare for the torch run."

"And what are other people telling you?"

"Well, we have a seventeen-year-old kid who is working out with ankle weights to build up his strength, and we have a woman who is jogging every day. What's your story?"

I laughed. "I guess mine would be a little unique." Then I told her about my arthritis and the scooter and the upcoming test run. She asked if they could bring out a crew. I was a bit hesitant—*What if I pull an Evel Knievel or something? I don't want that on the nightly news!*—but I also realized that it would be great publicity for my sponsors, to whom I owed so much.

"Sure," I said. "We'd love to have you."

The next day Channel 4 showed up with cameras in tow. They taped the assembling of the torch holder, which took almost five hours, and the test run that followed. I held the torch carefully, slid it into the holder, climbed onto the scooter, and started the engine. As everyone cheered, I slowly pulled away. Two minutes later, I came to a stop. The torch was still in place; my body was in one piece. I thought to myself, *Let's hope it goes this smoothly in two weeks.*

On April 27, 1996, the morning of the Olympic Torch Relay, I woke early, jolted out of bed by a combination of anxiety and excitement. In the preceding days, publicity surrounding the event had escalated. I was invited to appear on the nationally syndicated *Home and Family* television show. And there were several stories in the Asian press, which pointed out, with an understandable degree of agitation, that I was the only person of Asian descent in all of Los Angeles who had been asked to participate in the relay. As I thought about this, the butterflies took flight in my stomach. I walked to the window of my bedroom, opened the curtains, and let the warmth of the California sun splash across my face. It was a perfect day.

My entire family came down to L.A. for the event. We had decided ahead of time that they would all wear the same color clothing, so that I'd be able to spot them in the crowd. Because red is my favorite color (and because it's considered a lucky color in Chinese culture), they all wore red polo shirts. We went out for Chinese dim sum in the morning, and then they dropped me off at an organizational meeting for the torchbearers. For three hours we received instructions on basic protocol: how to carry the torch properly, what to do, what not to do. Then we went off to our designated spots along the torch route.

The relay started in the Los Angeles Coliseum. Four hours later, accompanied by an entourage approximately six blocks long, it arrived in Hollywood, where I was stationed. The sidewalks were packed with people screaming and applauding. I saw familiar friends with signs that read "Go, Bionic Babe!" and "Scoot, Amye, Scoot!" I'd never seen anything like it. A local television sportscaster ran the leg prior to mine. As he drew near, I could see a broad smile on his face. We hugged, and he passed me the torch. Actually, each of the participants in the relay has his own torch; it's the *flame* that is passed. The tips of our torches kissed, and mine burst into fire. Moments later, his would be extinguished and I would be the temporary guardian of the Olympic spirit.

With great care I placed the torch in the torch holder. Then I climbed onto the scooter and drove away. I was so full of adrenaline that it was hard to maintain a slow, steady pace. There were people all around me: four policemen on motorcycles, a camera crew, two Olympic officials, and a bunch of other people I didn't even recognize. As I glanced over my shoulder I was stunned to see my seventy-year-old mother jogging behind me, along with little Amye and Nick and Christopher. I had no idea they were going to do that. They kept yelling "Go, Amye!"

For six-tenths of a mile we went on like that, as if in slow motion. To my right was a sidewalk clotted with people standing three deep. To my left was the Hollywood Freeway. Traffic here usually zips along at a frightening pace, but now it resembled a parking lot, as people leaned on their horns and shouted encouragement: "Go, America!" "Yeah, keep on going, babe!"

It's amazing what you remember, the snapshots that linger in your mind. I can still see a man standing on the sidewalk, holding a tiny baby aloft, reaching out plaintively, as if he wanted me to anoint the child or something. I felt like I was the Pope! It was funny, in a way, but it was also extraordinarily moving, this feeling of national pride and unconditional support. The sight of the Olympic torch has that sort of effect on people.

The beginning of each leg of the relay was marked by a purple flag. As I approached the end of my segment, I could see the flag waving, and beside it I could see the next torchbearer smiling and jogging in place. We touched torches and his flame ignited. Then he gave me a big high-five and a hug, and off he went. The final step was to extinguish the flame on my torch, a simple matter for most people, but virtually impossible for me. I tried to turn the small knob on the bottom of the torch that controlled the flow of butane, but my fingers weren't strong enough. We had been told at the meeting, "If you have any problems at all, don't panic; just defer to your escorts." So that's what I did, and they handled the situation wonderfully. As the procession rumbled away, the flame on my torch flickered and died. My part was over.

Before I had time to take it all in, someone grabbed my scooter and I was whisked away to a waiting bus, which was filled with all the other torchbearers. They applauded as I climbed aboard and then we began hugging and shaking hands. It was like being part of an athletic team, a thrilling, communal experience I hadn't known since high school. The sweet irony, of course, was that I was able to participate not only in spite of my arthritis, but because of it.

The bus trailed behind the caravan for the next mile or two. We picked up a few more torchbearers and then broke off to return to the designated drop-off point. An enthusiastic mob greeted us— dozens of friends and family for each of the torchbearers. One of the first people I spotted was my father, whom I hadn't seen since that morning. Dad hadn't run alongside the scooter, so I had sort of lost track of him. Now, here he was, his arms extended, his eyes filled with tears. I thought about how far we had come, about all we had been through, and I started to cry, too.

Afterward my family took me to Wolfgang Puck's restaurant for pizza. My first inclination was to leave the torch (which I was allowed to keep as a souvenir) in our van, but my father blanched at that idea. "No!" he said. "Someone might steal it." So I walked into the restaurant with the smoldering torch in my hands. As the door closed behind me, the place fell silent. Everyone dropped their forks and stared. Within seconds we were approached by the manager.

"Is that the Olympic torch?" he asked, his eyes wide in disbelief. "Did you carry it?"

I nodded.

Suddenly I was surrounded by people I had never met. They all wanted to shake my hand, hold the torch. One woman asked if I would pose for a picture with her son. It was very strange, almost unnerving, as if there were some sort of mystical aura surrounding the torch, an inexplicable power to heal and cleanse and captivate. Who knows? Maybe there was. When I was interviewed by the local media that day, a reporter asked me, "Amye, did you feel any pain?"

I had to think about it for a moment. The question was simple, the answer complicated.

"I knew that pain was there," I said, "but I didn't care," That was the truth, too. I had been so exhilarated by the event that the pain simply didn't matter. In essence, I did not feel pain. For a brief, beautiful time—perhaps for the first time in my adult life—I was completely free.

14

Part of the Solution,
Not Part of the Problem

*Sometimes we fail to see that when a door closes . . . there is always a
window that opens.*

ALEXANDER GRAHAM BELL

For many years I kept that quote on my refrigera-
tor, affixed unceremoniously by a little magnet. Though small and
unobtrusive, it held a place of honor in both my home and heart,
for I saw it several times a day and repeated it almost as a mantra.
Those words helped sustain me in the deepest, darkest hours of my
illness, when I wondered what would become of my life, and how I
would survive the sentence I had been handed, a sentence of permanent disability and dependence.

Following my tenth joint replacement, early in the 1990s, I remember that my mother came to Los Angeles to help me in my
postoperative recovery, as she did after each of my surgical procedures. When it was time for her to return to her own life and her
own household and family, I felt a surge of panic and sadness unlike anything I had experienced in several years. I had walked into
my bedroom closet one evening to get a few things, with Mom trail-
ing behind. I moved slowly, awkwardly, and when I tried to flip on

the lights, and found it difficult because my newly repaired elbow was still inflamed, Mom was right there to help. It wasn't a big deal—she'd done things small and large for me countless times over the years, and this visit was no different. For some reason, though, the reality of the situation—the fact that I would periodically need assistance with the most mundane of tasks, probably for the rest of my life—settled in with new weight, and I began to cry. I looked at my mother and realized the day would come when she would not be able to help me through the trauma of surgery, and I wondered how I would cope. The stark fear of not having this support system—not having the woman who had wiped my rear end as a baby, and who had occasionally wiped my rear end as an adult because of severe arthritis—was paralytic. Surgical management and slavish devotion to medication was transforming me into an increasingly functional human being, but I knew that it was all temporary, that unless a cure was found, I'd have to endure another cycle of joint replacements years down the road . . . and my mother would not be there to help.

And that scared me to death.

It dawned on me that evening that I'd been dependent on so many people to arrive at this point, that the kindness and love of friends and family and casual acquaintances had combined to provide me with the wings to fly (metaphorically and relatively speaking, of course). But because so much of my life was about bionic parts that had a clearly defined shelf life, and because someday I'd be without the nucleus of my support system, I understood with new clarity the degree to which my work had only just begun. I had to devote more energy and time to the job I was doing in the arthritis community, because that job would not be complete until I felt secure in the knowledge that my life, and the lives of countless others, would not be dependent on the next joint-replacement surgery. In sum, I would not rest until a cure had been found for arthritis.

○   ○   ○

Since that time, doors have been closing and windows have been opening with some frequency; on the good days, and I'm happy to report there have been many of them in recent years, it seems as though doors and windows are opening at the same time. While I still rely on heavy doses of medication to calm my arthritis, and there are times when a flare puts me flat on my back for a while, I no longer rely on wheelchairs or crutches to get around. Gone, too, are the days when I relied on disability checks to pay my bills. Ironically, the disease that nearly robbed me of my will to live has now provided me an opportunity to earn a living as a motivational speaker and health consultant. The work has become my passion, and I am grateful for the chance to make a difference in this world.

In 1999, I received a phone call that led to another such opportunity. The man on the other end, Armin Kuder, a mentor and friend through the Arthritis Foundation, asked if I'd be interested in giving a speech. Now, I receive many such calls; in fact, the last five years of my life have been all about picking up the phone and hearing someone say, "We've heard of you and we've heard about your story, and we'd like you to share it with our audience for motivation, education, and advocacy." This time the call came from a friend who was on the International Steering Committee of the Bone and Joint Decade, a United Nations and World Health Organization–endorsed initiative that would begin in the year 2000 and go through 2010. The object: to increase global awareness about the need for research, education, and patient empowerment in the battle against diseases of the musculoskeletal system, including arthritis.

The international launch of the Bone and Joint Decade would take place in January of 2000, in Geneva, Switzerland. The purpose of this call was to solicit my services as a speaker. I actually balked a little at first, thinking, quite reasonably, that Geneva would be a cold and slippery city in January; quickly, however, I came to my senses and saw this as a tremendous opportunity. A trip to Geneva, one of the most beautiful cities in the world, is pretty exciting in itself, and the actual event, the commencement of a global initiative dealing with something that has consumed my adult life, sounded mighty intriguing.

So, accompanied by my mother (not so much as a medical assistant anymore but as a guest and companion), I flew to Geneva a few months later with the idea that I'd give a little speech, do some shopping, and keep my ears open to the possibility that the Bone and Joint Decade might develop into something clear and meaningful. Little did I realize that this was a major international gathering of four hundred representatives from some thirty countries that had already endorsed the concept of the Bone and Joint Decade. The schedule for the conference included an international press conference, at which I was to be one of the featured speakers (as the designated patient representative); a meeting of eminent scientists and physicians from around the world discussing epidemiology—trying to determine, specifically, what we knew about the burden of all these various diseases in the year 2000 so that we could create a baseline measure for future comparison; and, finally, a black-tie reception.

The reception, a regal affair hosted at the elegant President Wilson Hotel along Lake Geneva, included the presentation of a giant cake adorned with Roman candles and sparklers, fireworks literally shooting off the surface. Professor Lars Lidgren, M.D., Ph.D., from Sweden, chairman of the International Steering Committee, asked me to take part in cutting the cake. There we were, physician and patient advocate standing together, working together to launch an international initiative. I couldn't help but feel, as the flashbulbs popped and the crowd cheered, that this was the beginning of something truly worthwhile and important. I also thought, *How odd. Not too long ago I was someone who couldn't even bring a fork to her mouth. Now, I am standing in a beautiful ballroom in Geneva, Switzerland, representing patients from all over the world, surrounded by brilliant scientists and surgeons. How did this happen?*

Within a few months, Karsten Dreinhöfer, director of development who was also an orthopedic surgeon and health economist in Germany, visited me in California to discuss my involvement with the Bone and Joint Decade; they wanted me to be their spokesperson. It wasn't necessary for the handsome Dr. Dreinhöfer to take three days out of his busy schedule to recruit my services; I would have agreed over the phone. But in person, we had the chance to discuss the Decade's goals, how they hoped to achieve them, and the realities and challenges of an international initiative. By May 2000, I was named spokesperson and director of strategic relations. My work was now in the international arena.

After so many dark days and so much pain, after years spent counseling other arthritis patients who felt as though no one cared about their plight, I can't tell you how encouraging all this was. In addition to providing much-needed organization and resources for the war against arthritis and other musculoskeletal diseases and injuries, the Bone and Joint Decade sends a clear message to all of us who have been tormented by these illnesses: "You are not alone. You are not alone in your city or your country. You are not alone on this planet."

The Bone and Joint Decade is not only an aggressive step toward finding a cure for arthritis and other musculoskeletal disorders; it is also an acknowledgment that this is a global issue. There are hundreds of millions of people experiencing problems similar to those that I've experienced, and if we don't do something about it, this is going to be a major worldwide epidemic. The amount of money that I alone have needed to tap into the medical system and to pay for my surgeries is not an insignificant amount. Multiply it by a million, or ten million, or one hundred million, and you have a financial, political, and emotional drain that few societies could withstand. The concept behind the Bone and Joint Decade is to re-duce the burden of these disorders on society, families, and people like Amye Leong. I know now that there is an army of talented, car-ing people out there who are willing to work with me to achieve this goal. At the same time, the realization that there is a global aspect to this disease reinforces what I have always believed: that arthritis transcends traditional boundaries of language, geography, and cul-ture. How many people in other countries are going through exactly what I've gone through? And how many of them, like that elderly woman I met in mainland China, don't have access to the care that I've been fortunate to have? When I think of that my blood boils and I become more resolute in my work as an advocate. I think of all the challenges I've been through, all the painful days, the awkward interactions with people who don't seem to understand or care, and I imagine multiplying that by millions, and the problem seems overwhelming, the obstacles almost insurmountable.

What the Bone and Joint Decade really represents is hope, for there can be no chance of victory without first admitting the scope of the struggle. Rather than being against me, against *us*, the forces are coming to our assistance: the United Nations; the World Health Organization; the World Bank; over 750 professional rheumatology, orthopedic, and rehabilitation societies; patient advocacy organi-zations; even the Pope! Pharmaceutical companies are now initiat-ing patient-oriented education and empowerment programs like the Patient Advisory Council by Aventis and the Patient Partner program by Pharmacia—and supporting national and global ef-forts like the Bone and Joint Decade. They're on my team now and I am on theirs. That's very exciting.

One of the more encouraging recent developments in the cam-paign to increase public awareness of arthritis is the active in-volvement of people with instant name recognition. One example is, Joe Montana, the former quarterback for the San Francisco 49ers. In winning all those Super Bowl rings and Most Valuable Player trophies, Montana assured himself of a spot in the Pro Football Hall of Fame. He also forfeited the right to be a healthy, active middle-aged man. I had an opportunity to speak with Joe not long ago, when we both addressed Congress about the value of arthritis research, and he told me that he has developed such severe osteoarthritis in his knees—the cost of taking thousands of punishing blows from three-hundred-pound linemen—that he can't even play pickup basketball with his own children. I had asked him, "When did you know it was really bad?"

Joe pursed his lips. "Amye," he said, "football is my game. Everybody knows that. But my real love is basketball. Always has been. One day, while I was dropping my two girls off at basketball practice, I noticed they didn't have enough people to scrimmage; they were one person short. *No problem*, I thought. *I'll help out.* Guess what? I could barely get up and down the court. I couldn't keep up with a bunch of junior high school girls, my knees were so inflamed. That's when it hit me: *I'm barely forty-five years old, and I'm an old man!*"

Joe related another story about how he and his wife were sitting in the front row during the 49ers seventy-fifth anniversary celebration, watching as dozens of former players were introduced. All were world-famous, gifted, powerful athletes who, in their prime, could do almost anything on the football field. Now they were paying the price for their glory. One by one they heard their names, stood, and took small, slow, awkward steps across the stage. Some could barely walk at all.

"I watched these guys, many of whom were my teammates," Joe Montana recalled, "and I thought, *'If I don't do something, that's going to be me in a few years.'* "

So Joe is *my* teammate now, and I find that to be at once ironic and exciting. Here is a guy who had an aura of invincibility, and now he's suffering from chronic arthritis pain and drastically reduced mobility. I'm grateful for Joe's involvement; the more we can recruit well-known people affected by arthritis, the better. I've had the unique pleasure of working with celebrities like Victoria Principal, Frankie Avalon, Mickey Gilley, and Sarah Purcell in the arthritis cause. There is, in fact, a role for everyone. Governments become involved because they realize the cost of this disease is exorbitant, and preventing disability saves lives and money. The corporate world becomes involved for very practical reasons: the arthritis population represents a pervasive market. There is a role for every person, family, institution, company, and government that wants to put an end to the disability caused by arthritis.

We've come a long way in the last quarter century, from a time when the Arthritis Foundation swam solitarily upstream, offering support for people with arthritis but getting little or no support in return from the federal government. In the 1980s a sufficient number of influential people got together and said, "We need more," and thus was born in 1985 the National Institute of Arthritis, Musculoskeletal and Skin Disease. That was great, but NIAMS was given a minuscule budget, not nearly enough to adequately serve the millions of people under its umbrella. It wasn't until people with arthritis, along with surgeons and scientists and rheumatologists, stood up and made their voices heard that the crumbs of funding became cookies. Under the leadership of Dr. Steven Katz, NIAMS has risen in its level of importance and visibility. The U.S. Centers for Disease Control and Prevention has taken a leadership role in funding community-based education programs around the nation. Congress, which dictates the level of program funding, is slowly beginning to see that an investment in arthritis research and education is a major step toward preventing pain, suffering, and disability. But we still need more. More money and more voices, more people saying, "How come there isn't enough money to help to find a cure for this disease that cripples my husband . . . my daughter . . . my father . . . my grandmother? Why don't you *care?*"

∘ ∘ ∘

In the spring of 2000, the United States, under the Clinton administration, became the twenty-fifth nation to declare its support for the Bone and Joint Decade. I wish we had been the first, but I'm nonetheless pleased that we've acknowledged the importance of this initiative, for when the richest and most powerful country in the world gets involved, everything changes.

Under the leadership of national coordinator, Dr. Stuart Weinstein, and with the help of the American Academy of Orthopaedic Surgeons, fifty-six musculoskeletal patient-advocacy and health-professional organizations launched the Bone and Joint Decade in the United States with a luncheon at the Willard Hotel in Washington, D.C. The president offered his support in a communiqué:

THE WHITE HOUSE
WASHINGTON
MAY 26, 2000

Warm greetings to everyone observing 2000 to 2010 as the Bone and Joint Decade.

One out of every four Americans suffers from a musculoskeletal condition caused by injury or disease—a condition that often places difficult emotional and financial burdens on patients and their families. Affecting people of all ages, these conditions are the most common causes of severe long-term pain and physical disability for people around the world. In the United States alone, musculoskeletal conditions result in more than 131 million patient visits to health-care providers each year.

I commend the many volunteers, professionals, and patient-advocacy organizations who are devoting their time and energy to increasing awareness of the seriousness and widespread impact of musculoskeletal diseases and injuries. Through your efforts to im-

prove prevention, treatment, and rehabilitation, your commitment to research, and your participation in a variety of Bone and Joint Decade activities, you are bringing hope to countless people around the world and helping to create a brighter, healthier future for us all.

Best wishes for a successful observance.

BILL CLINTON

Some of the people in that room had devoted their entire professional lives to arthritis advocacy, and had waited thirty years or more to hear something like this. I had been working for more than twenty years to get my body well enough to walk into that room without mechanical assistance, to reach a point where people would say, "Wow, you don't look like you have arthritis!" So to hear these words of encouragement and support coming directly from the White House, well, my reaction was . . . *It's about time!*

Not long after that, Dr. Weinstein stepped to the podium to introduce one of the luncheon's featured speakers: me. Part of the introduction was a three-minute video, produced by the Arthritis Foundation, in which Amye Leong's life story, at least as it relates to arthritis, is neatly and graphically summarized. Projected on a twelve-foot screen were pictures of a waiflike girl in a wheelchair, then on crutches. There were grisly close-ups of my deformed toes taken before surgery, and more close-ups afterward, when the toes were replaced by swollen, purple lumps of flesh skewered by tiny metal rods. The tape rolled on, filling the room with stark and grim shots of a woman seemingly sentenced to a life of pain and suffering. The final image was a freeze-frame of the woman in physical therapy exercising her withered arms, and somehow managing to smile through it all.

The video ended, the lights came up, and there was the crippled woman in the video walking across the stage, moving without assistance of any kind. The reaction, a low murmur that grew into thunderous applause, was something that can best be described as enthusiastic disbelief. *This can't be the same woman? Can it?*

"It's a pleasure to be standing here before you," I began. "Fifteen years ago, I couldn't have done this. I'm so lucky to have had the opportunities I've had, to have been blessed with so many friends and such a wonderful, supportive family. I'm lucky to have had the tools necessary for withstanding and enduring this torture."

I don't believe in shrinking from the reality of arthritis; I don't see any reason to paint a pretty picture for my audience, or to spare them the graphic details. That's false and misleading and serves no purpose. And so I talked about the wonderful meal they were being served that day, and the pleasure of eating, the sights and smells and tastes, and the long period of my life when eating was an act of humiliation, because I relied on my mother and father to hand-feed me. I wanted them to understand and appreciate something as simple as picking up a knife and fork, because for many with arthritis, looking at a fork is like looking at a gaping chasm.

"Thanks to research, I am able to be here today," I went on. "But my future is tied to joint-replacement surgeries, because unless we find a cure, I'm going to have to go through this all over again. To be perfectly candid, I don't know that I can afford it—spiritually, emotionally, financially. I may look perfectly fine, but I'm still deteriorating. The disease is still active. This disease is still eating me from the inside out.

"This day—and what it represents—is important to me, and it should be important to every person in this room, because you represent the organizations and governments that have the ability to make finding a cure a reality. We all have to fight for a little more money, a little more support, and a *lot* more publicity. That stack of grant proposals sitting on your desk? Who knows? Maybe a cure is sitting in one of those. So keep looking, keep fighting, keep trying."

I ended my talk with an assertion that although we have made progress, we are not yet close to winning the war. Over the clinking and clattering of silverware and china, I implored them, "Every time you pick up a fork, please think of the woman in that video. Think of the millions of people like her, people who cannot eat, and who may not have a mother around to feed them.

"Thank you."

The response was more than I could have hoped for, heartfelt applause and cheers that raised goose bumps on my arms. I left the stage and took my seat, right next to a woman named Dr. Dorothy Rice, an esteemed health economist whose talk provided hard statistics about the burden of disease. Dorothy, a distinguished and elegant woman, leaned over and took my hands in hers.

"You," she said, "are the reason I do my work."

I smiled and thanked her. And with the room still shaking, the ovation rolling on, I added, "We all have our part in this, don't we?"

15

Dream Come True

Like all teenagers, I grew up with aspirations and dreams. One dream was to live and study French in Paris. Something about all the pictures I had seen of Paris exuded a sense of style, romance, sophistication, and passion. I was drawn to it with excitement. But when rheumatoid arthritis invaded my life, all my dreams went out the window. My life was consumed first by its devastation, and then by years of surgery and rehabilitation so that I could regain the simple, everyday functions that were lost to the ravages of joint disease.

In June 2000, just a few months into my new position as spokesperson of the Bone and Joint Decade, I found myself walking along the Seine River in Paris. After business meetings in London, I met my girlfriend Jessica Saal, and we headed for the French capital for a few days. The sight of Notre Dame and the gaiety of the people walking the stone sidewalks sparked in me the memory of a dream once lost.

As Jessica and I talked and laughed, I suddenly stopped and announced, "Jess, I can actually see myself living here. Oh my gosh! That was a dream I had when I was a kid. I almost forgot about it altogether."

"Do you know anyone who lives here?" Jess asked.

"No . . . not yet," I quipped with an eerie sense of optimism.

After four glorious days of seeing the beauty of Paris, we arrived back home in California, but the images of the city were stuck in my mind.

Could I actually live there, given my arthritis needs? Paris is an old city and not very accessible for people with mobility problems. I don't even speak the language, even though I love its sound. How would I get the things I need?

Through years of learning to live with arthritis, I had become an expert problem solver. Don't panic. Get the facts, all the facts, before making any kind of decision. Weigh all the evidence. Talk with the experts, people who have had real experience. Ask questions with a childlike curiosity. Set realistic goals. Set milestones to pave the way for progress and advancement. Advocate for what you believe. Take progress notes. And reward yourself for achieving the milestones with things that bring you joy. Most important of all, lighten up! Don't be so serious. And, finally, breathe. These strategies had gotten me through the darkest days of arthritis and years of relearning how to walk and to reach with my arms all over again. Could these same strategies work in determining if I could live in a foreign country?

For the next five months, I spoke with and e-mailed friends, acquaintances, health professionals, even relative strangers. I sought out anyone who had lived in Paris. I kept a journal to document names, their experiences, and their references. A passion for exploration about all things Parisian became my hobby.

Through my arthritis journey, I have come to believe in the connected nature of the universe, in the way that opportunities present themselves to us at precisely the right times in our lives. Call it fate if you like. Associations and resources would pop up at times when I thought I didn't want them, but in fact needed them. And this Paris exploration was no different.

Back in California, I was interviewed by the *International Herald Tribune* for a story on international business travel by people with disabilities. Through my work with the Bone and Joint Decade, I had become quite familiar with transatlantic flying in a few short months. The story appeared in their weekly travel column and quoted me, citing my position and my challenges with arthritis. Within a few days, I received an e-mail from a gentleman named Peter Kenton, an attorney who was interested in learning how I had become a motivational speaker despite living with the uncertainties of arthritis. Peter, a longtime resident of Paris, inquired if we could ever get together. *Thank you, universe!*

Making a move to Paris is no small effort, particularly if you don't yet speak the language. It's not as if you can just pick up a newspaper to find an apartment. Through my friendship with Peter, I became acquainted with his friend, a lovely woman named Anna Eicher, who owns a consulting company specializing in helping people find housing in Paris. Although she typically deals with companies transferring employees overseas, she consented to take me on as an individual client. Through the thousands of miles and the nine-hour difference between California and France, Anna helped me identify the kind of amenities I would need in an apartment. Once I signed a contract to use Anna's services, I was committed to making Paris my home. There was no looking back.

I had spoken to my rheumatologist, Dr. Elaine Lambert of Palo Alto, and to my orthopedic surgeon, Dr. Christopher Mow of Stanford Medical Center. Initially, they seemed enthusiastic about my dream, but they also questioned my ability to maintain the medical care to which I had become accustomed: monthly office visits to regulate my medications; regular X rays to note bone and joint changes, and recommend orthotics to help ease the pain of walk-ing; regulating my range-of-motion and strengthening exercise rou-tine to maintain my mobility. Keeping me moving takes an army of dedicated professionals and friends. Yet I was becoming even more obsessed about trying to make my dream a reality and my doctors agreed to help me. With their assistance, via e-mail and references to other health professionals in Paris, this could actually work.

By March 2001, Mom and I were flying to Paris with the explicit goal of finding Amye just the right apartment. Mom had been through so much with me and had given up so much to take care of me. Having her accompany me, to find an apartment and see Paris for the very first time, was a small token of gratitude to her. Thanks to Anna, we hit Paris running. Anna escorted us through apartment after apartment. Because of arthritis, my requirements were pretty strict: no more than two blocks from the Metro (since I wasn't plan-ning to have a car in Paris); at least two elevators (in case one broke); accessible cupboards and bathrooms; lots of closet space; room for an in-home office; and a view, of course . . . all within my price range!

On our fourth day in Paris (only twenty-four hours before re-turning to California), I was growing somber. Nothing had really stood out in terms of my perfect space. Maybe this wasn't meant to be. That evening, as we were getting ready for dinner, we heard whooping and singing beneath our window. We were staying at the lovely Notre Dame Hotel, located just across the street from the magnificent cathedral in Rive Gauche. We opened our windows to the street just in time to see hundreds of people on Rollerblades streaming down the streets of Paris. As they passed through the in-tersection of our hotel, the roar of the rolling crowd floated upward, as if to proclaim victory about a passion for life itself. It was infec-tious. From our third story window, Mom and I hollered back, "Ya-hoooo . . . c'est la vie!"

That night, with both Leong women tucked into their beds after yet another fabulous Parisian meal, I settled in to read the latest edition of *FUSAC*, a French-U.S. paper filled with classified advertising. I was still determined to find an apartment. So I serendipitously opened the newspaper to a midsection page. A tiny ad jumped out at me as if to bite me on the nose: *16th arrondissement, 2 bedrooms, 2 baths, balconies, view of Eiffel Tower.* It sounded great, and it was cheaper than the apartment I had almost settled on taking. I rose up out of bed and shook Mom.

"Mom, Mom, listen to this," I said, nudging her out of a deep sleep. I read the ad out loud and got a sigh for a response.

"Yeah, Amye."

"I'm going to call on this first thing in the morning. Do you think we're too late?" Mom was already fast asleep. I crawled back under my covers and imagined what the apartment might be like as I drifted off into a deep sleep.

A beautiful morning sun greeted us on our last day in Paris. In the previous four days, Anna had taken us to more than a dozen apartments. But my intuition drove me to call on this particular apartment right away and not wait for Anna's help, so I dialed the telephone number listed. I had come to rely so much on Anna that I forgot that her expertise and facility with the French language made our work seem so easy. When I got an answering machine with a woman's voice speaking French, I bit my lip. What do I say? Would she understand my English? I introduced myself, gave my professional background, and asked to see the apartment this morning, explaining that we were returning to the United States in the afternoon. Within an hour, a sophisticated woman named Caroline returned my call and invited us to visit the apartment at noon.

At precisely noon, Anna and her daughter, Alexandria, Mom, and I were greeted at the street door of the apartment building by Caroline. The minute we walked into the apartment, I knew it was "the one." With antique furniture, original artwork on the walls, Chinese and Persian carpets throughout, the apartment had the feel of home. As Caroline escorted us into the bathroom, I noticed a long cord hanging on the wall by the bathtub.

"May I ask you what this is for?" I inquired.

Caroline explained that the apartment was owned by a woman whose family had recently put her into an assisted-living center— because of her severe arthritis. The cord was to call for help from the bathtub. Mom's mouth dropped open, my eyes nearly popped, and we chuckled together. When Caroline asked if we were all right, I explained that I worked for an international health organization that helps people with musculoskeletal disorders like arthritis, that I was crippled by the disease as a young adult and had since gone through many joint replacements to walk and function again. Caroline smiled.

"Well, my dear, then this apartment is perfect for you."

I made the transatlantic move to Paris in May 2001. Every evening, as I go out on my balcony to take in the beauty of the City of Lights and stand in amazement at the sight of the Eiffel Tower aglow in amber lights, I think back to those days of being confined to a wheelchair. I recall Mom feeding me, Dad reconstructing their Bakersfield home to accommodate their disabled daughter, the professors who told me to go home because I was too sick to stay in graduate school, and the hundreds of nights spent in hospitals thinking my life was over. Because of crippling arthritis, my dreams were nearly taken away. But today, because of my work in arthritis and musculoskeletal disorders, my dream of living in Paris has come alive. How long I've waited for this moment.

So please, remember, dreams can come true.

RESOURCES

Websites

Access to quality information is the bedrock of making good decisions about managing any aspect of arthritis. The following resources can make a world of difference for you. But be aware:

- Websites constantly go in and out of business and their content is constantly changing.
- Websites know no geographical bounds, so don't let your nationalistic thinking prevent you from seeking information from the global community of virtual information. Check out information from international sources.
- Approach resource information like a detective: Look at the source of the information for credibility; look at the credentials of the authors for expertise and experience; look at the date of the information to ensure the most up-to-date piece; and check out who sponsors the website, as this may color the information provided.
- Be aware of any hidden messages in the information, for example, the marketing of one product over others.

In today's age of technology, I highly recommend that you invest in a computer and Internet service provider. Being able to sit within the comfort of your own home to scan the virtual universe of information is convenient and easy, and will cause less wear and tear on your body. Access to a computer terminal and the Internet is also a mainstay of most libraries. The information highway is at your fingertips, so let your fingers do the walking. Happy hunting!

ORGANIZATIONS

The arthritis patient organizations and not-for-profit websites represent and address the needs of people affected by the many forms of arthritis in their respective countries. Generally, they provide information, education, advocacy, and support services. Becoming a member of the patient organization in your country will help you become connected to the many services offered and the opportunities to make a difference for yourself and others in a similar position. It is through these organizations that I have met enduring lifelong friends. I hope you will find a similar experience.

ARTHRITIS FOUNDATION (UNITED STATES)
www.arthritis.org

CANADIAN ARTHRITIS SOCIETY
www.arthritis.ca

ARTHRITIS CARE (UNITED KINGDOM)
www.arthritiscare.org.uk

ARTHRITIS FOUNDATION OF IRELAND
www.arthritis-foundation.com

ARTHRITIS FOUNDATION OF AUSTRALIA
www.arthritisfoundation.com.au

ARTHRITIS FOUNDATION OF NEW ZEALAND
www.arthritis.org.nz

ARTHRITIS INSIGHT
www.arthritisinsight.com

OSTERREICHISCHE RHEUMALIGA (AUSTRIAN RHEUMATISM LEAGUE)
www.rheumaliga.at

ASSOCIATION FRANÇAISE DE LUTTE ANTIRHUMATISMALE (ASSOCIATION OF FRENCH LEAGUES AGAINST RHEUMATISM)
www.aflar.unice.fr

DANISH RHEUMATISM ASSOCIATION
www.gigtforeningen.dk

DEUTSCHE RHEUMA LIGA (GERMAN RHEUMATISM LEAGUE)
www.rheuma-liga.de

FINNISH RHEUMATISM ASSOCIATION
www.reumaliitto.fi

ICELANDIC LEAGUE AGAINST RHEUMATISM
www.gigt.is

JAPAN RHEUMATISM FOUNDATION (IN JAPANESE ONLY)
www.rheuma-net.or.jp

LATVIAN LEAGUE AGAINST RHEUMATISM
www.gigt.is

LIGA REUMATÓGICA ESPANOLA (SPANISH LEAGUE AGAINST RHEUMATISM)
www.lire.es

NATIONAL ARTHRITIS FOUNDATION OF SINGAPORE
www.arthritis.org.sg

NORSK REVMATIKERFORBUND (NORWEGIAN RHEUMATISM ASSOCIATION)
www.rheuma.no

NORDIC RHEUMA COUNCIL
www.nrr.nu

PEOPLE WITH ARTHRITIS/RHEUMATISM IN EUROPE
www.paremanifesto.org

PORTUGUESE LEAGUE AGAINST RHEUMATISM
www.lpcdr.pt

REUMATIKERFÖRBUNDET (SWEDISH RHEUMATISM ASSOCIATION)
www.reumatikerforbundet.org

SWISS LEAGUE AGAINST RHEUMATISM
www.rheumaliga.ch

SWISS POLYARTHRITIS ASSOCIATION
www.arthritis.ch

A Special Word about the Arthritis Foundation: The Arthritis Foundation (U.S.) is the most comprehensive arthritis patient organization in the world. With chapter offices in nearly every state, it offers a wide variety of relevant and up-to-date information; an award-winning bimonthly magazine called *Arthritis Today;* and local programs that really do make a difference in the daily management of arthritis, such as symposia, exercise classes, advocacy summits, and young adult and children's programs. It takes a proactive role in advocating for the needs of people with arthritis and a leadership role in urging increased funding for arthritis research. Because of its commitment to funding rheumatology training, we have seen the number of quality rheumatologists increase to meet the treatment needs of people with arthritis. Unique to its organizational management is the role those affected by arthritis play in participating in the policy development and leadership of individual chapters and at the national level. I urge you to get to know the Arthritis Foundation in your area and get involved. Log on to their website, call (800) 283-7800, or check the telephone book for the number of your local chapter.

Children and Young Adults

AMERICAN JUVENILE ARTHRITIS ORGANIZATION
www.arthritis.org/communities/children_young_adults.asp

BRAVE KIDS
www.bravekids.org

DANISH ORGANISATION OF YOUTH WITH RHEUMATISM (DANISH AND ENGLISH)
www.fnug.dk

DANISH PARENTS ASSOCIATION OF CHILDREN WITH ARTHRITIS (DANISH AND ENGLISH)
www.gbf.dk/enghome.html

INTERNATIONAL ORGANISATION OF YOUTH WITH RHEUMATISM (IOYR)
www.ioyr.org

INTERNATIONAL STILL'S DISEASE FOUNDATION
www.stillsdisease.org

JRA WORLD
http://jraworld.arthritisinsight.com

Ankylosing Spondylitis

SPONDYLITIS ASSOCIATION OF AMERICA
www.spondylitis.org

NATIONAL ANKYLOSING SPONDYLITIS SOCIETY (UNITED KINGDOM)
www.nass.co.uk

Fibromyalgia

AMERICAN FIBROMYALGIA SYNDROME ASSOCIATION
www.afsafund.org

FIBROMYALGIA ASSOCIATION UNITED KINGDOM
www.UKFibromyalgia.com

NATIONAL FIBROMYALGIA AWARENESS CAMPAIGN
www.fmaware.com

USA FIBROMYALGIA ASSOCIATION
www.w2.com/fibro1.html

Lupus

LUPUS FOUNDATION OF AMERICA
www.lupus.org

LUPUS AUCKLAND
www.lupus.org.nz

LUPUS CANADA
www.lupuscanada.org

LUPUS HEALTHNET
www.lupusnet.ucalgary.ca

Osteoporosis

INTERNATIONAL OSTEOPOROSIS FOUNDATION
www.osteofound.org

LEBANESE OSTEOPOROSIS PREVENTION SOCIETY
www.lops.org

NATIONAL OSTEOPOROSIS FOUNDATION
www.nof.org

NATIONAL OSTEOPOROSIS SOCIETY (UNITED KINGDOM)
www.nos.org.uk

OSTEOPOROSIS AUSTRALIA
www.osteoporosis.org.au

OSTEOPOROSIS INTERNATIONAL
www.link.springerny.com/link/service/journals/00198/index.htm

OSTEOPOROSIS NEW ZEALAND
www.osteoporosis.org.nz

OSTEOPOROSIS SOCIETY OF CANADA
www.osteoporosis.ca

OSTEOPOROSIS SOCIETY OF THE PHILIPPINES
www.ospi.org.ph

Osteogenesis Imperfecta

OSTEOGENESIS IMPERFECTA FOUNDATION
www.oif.org

OSTEOGENESIS IMPERFECTA FEDERATION EUROPE
www.oife.org

Sjogren's Syndrome

SJOGREN'S SYNDROME FOUNDATION
www.sjogrens.org

BRITISH SJOGREN'S SYNDROME ASSOCIATION
www.ourworld.compuserve.com/homepages/bssassociation

NEW ZEALAND SJOGREN'S SYNDROME
www.dry.org/nz

SWEDISH SJOGREN'S SYNDROME ASSOCIATION
www.sjogrensyndrom.se

Scleroderma

SCLERODERMA FOUNDATION
www.scleroderma.org

SCLERODERMA RESEARCH FOUNDATION
www.srfcure.org

Psoriasis

NATIONAL PSORIASIS FOUNDATION
www.psoriasis.org

PSORIATIC ARTHOPATHY ALLIANCE
www.paalliance.org

GOVERNMENT ORGANIZATIONS

NATIONAL INSTITUTE OF ARTHRITIS AND MUSCULOSKELETAL AND SKIN DISEASES
www.niams.nih.gov
NIAMS is the primary branch of the U.S. National Institutes of Health, the mission of which is to support research into the causes, treatment, and prevention of arthritis and musculoskeletal and skin diseases. The NIAMS Office of Information Dissemination provides a quality variety of free educational booklets.

CENTERS FOR DISEASE CONTROL AND PREVENTION
www.cdc.gov
The CDC has taken a collaborative leadership approach to the prevention of arthritis in the U.S. The National Arthritis Action Plan (NAAP) is a comprehensive, coordinated strategy to address the rising epidemic of arthritis. The Arthritis Foundation and the Association of State and Territorial Health Officers play pivotal roles in the plan.

NATIONAL INSTITUTES OF HEALTH, OSTEOPOROSIS AND RELATED BONE DISEASES—
NATIONAL RESOURCE CENTER
www.osteo.org

HEALTHFINDER
www.healthfinder.gov

EDUCATIONAL INSTITUTIONS

JOHNS HOPKINS ARTHRITIS
www.hopkins-arthritis.som.jhmi.edu

MISSOURI ARTHRITIS REHABILITATION AND RESEARCH TRAINING CENTER
www.muhealth.org/~arthritis/index.html

MEDICAL COLLEGE OF WISCONSIN PHYSICIANS AND CLINICS
http://healthlink.mcw.edu/arthritis/

STUDY OF RHEUMATOID ARTHRITIS—DUQUESNE UNIVERSITY
www.duq.edu/PT/RA/RA.html

UNIVERSITY OF WASHINGTON DEPARTMENT OF ORTHOPAEDICS
www.orthop.washington.edu

CORPORATIONS

ABOUT ARTHRITIS
http://arthritis.about.com

HEALTHTALK INTERACTIVE—RHEUMATOID ARTHRITIS INFORMATION NETWORK
www.healthtalk.com/rain
In conjunction with the Washington Chapter Arthritis Foundation.

HEALING WELL—ARTHRITIS
www.healingwell.com/arthritis

INTELLIHEALTH—ARTHRITIS
www.intelihealth.com
Sponsored by Aetna featuring consumer health information from
Harvard Medical School.

RAACCESS
www.raaccess.com
Sponsored by Wyeth-Ayerst Pharmaceuticals and Immunex Corporation.

RAWATCH.COM
www.rawatch.com
Sponsored by Aventis Pharmaceuticals.

ARTHRITIS
www.arthritis.com

Sponsored by Pharmacia, this website is the second generation of ArthritisConnection.com.

MEDICINENET, INC.
www.medicinenet.com

CORPORATE-SPONSORED PROGRAMS

Patient Partners

PHARMACIA
Sponsored by Pharmacia, people with arthritis are certified to provide hands-on Physical Diagnosis of Arthritis (PDA) and a Musculoskeletal Rapid Screener to medical students or other health professionals. The program is being conducted in the United States, Europe, and Japan. Contact a Pharmacia representative through your physician for more information.

Patient Advisory Council

MEDICAL INFORMATION SERVICES, INC.
Originally sponsored by Aventis Pharmaceuticals in conjunction with the Arthritis Foundation (U.S.), thirteen individuals were selected from the prestigious "50 Heroes Overcoming Arthritis" campaign by the Arthritis Foundation. A patient-led movement, the original thirteen PAC members share their experiences with health professionals for wider dissemination through the newsletter, ImpactRA, and on video for education of managed care organizations and professionals to improve access and treatment of rheumatic diseases.

GENERAL HEALTH

U.S. NATIONAL LIBRARY OF MEDICINE
www.nlm.nih.gov/contacts/contact.html
This is the world's largest medical library and the creator of Medline, an on-line medical library search service.

COMBINED HEALTH INFORMATION DATABASE
www.chid.aerie.com
Produced by the National Institutes of Health, Centers for Disease Control and Prevention, and the Health Resources and Services Administration of

the U.S. Public Health Service, this database provides a host of health promotion and educational materials not indexed elsewhere.

JOHNS HOPKINS INFONET
www@infonet.welch.jhu.edu

PHYSICIAN'S DESK REFERENCE
www.pdr.net
The PDR has provided package insert information on drugs for years. This same information is now available online at a site that includes much more. Drug interactions, prices, and even herbal medications are covered. In addition, the site presents information for patients and other health professionals in an orderly and useful fashion.

CASE MANAGEMENT RESOURCE GUIDE
www.cmrg.com
This is a great patient guide to health-care resources. When you don't have access to a social worker to scan all the resources in your area, this guide gives you listings of what you'll need in any area of the United States—forty categories of health-care services and resources including home care, rehabilitation, long-term care, assisted living facilities, medical products manufacturers, and air medical transport.

JOURNALS

NEW ENGLAND JOURNAL OF MEDICINE
www.nejm.org

CANADIAN MEDICAL ASSOCIATION JOURNAL
www.cma.ca/cmaj/index.htm

JOURNAL OF AMERICAN MEDICAL ASSOCIATION
www.jama.com

ANNALS OF THE RHEUMATIC DISEASES
http://ard.bmjjournals.com

ARTHRITIS CARE AND RESEARCH
www.interscience.wiley.com/jpages/0004-3591+/

ARTHRITIS AND RHEUMATISM
www.interscience.wiley.com/jpages/0004-3591/

ARTHRITIS RESEARCH
www.interscience.wiley.com/jpages/0004-3591/

BEST PRACTICE & RESEARCH CLINICAL RHEUMATOLOGY
www.harcourt-international.com/journals/berh/default.cfm

BONE ONLINE
www.meddevel.com/site.mash?left=/library.exe&m1=1&m2=1&right=/library.exe&action=home&site=BONE&jcode=BON

CLINICAL RHEUMATOLOGY
http://link.springer-ny.com/link/service/journals/10067/index.htm

CURRENT OPINION IN RHEUMATOLOGY
www.co-rheumatology.com

JOINT BONE SPINE
www.jointbonespine.com

JOURNAL OF CLINICAL RHEUMATOLOGY
www.jclinrheum.com

JOURNAL OF RHEUMATOLOGY
www.jrheum.com

RHEUMATOLOGY
rheumatology.oupjournals.org

RHEUMATOLOGY & MUSCULOSKELETAL MEDICINE FOR PRIMARY CARE
www.rheumatology.org/publications/primarycare

RHEUMATOLOGY INTERNATIONAL
http://link.springer.de/link/service/journals/00296/index.htm

SCANDINAVIAN JOURNAL OF RHEUMATOLOGY
www.tandf.co.uk/journals/tfs/03009742.html

PROFESSIONAL SOCIETIES

AMERICAN COLLEGE OF RHEUMATOLOGY
www.rheumatology.org

ASSOCIATION OF RHEUMATOLOGY HEALTH PROFESSIONALS
www.rheumatology.org/arhp

EUROPEAN LEAGUE AGAINST RHEUMATISM
www.eular.org

INTERNATIONAL LEAGUE OF ASSOCIATIONS FOR RHEUMATOLOGY
www.ilar.org

CLINICAL TRIALS

NATIONAL INSTITUTES OF HEALTH CLINICAL TRIALS
www.clinicaltrials.gov

VERITAS MEDICINE
www.veritasmedicine.com/trial
This clinical trials database currently includes nineteen clinical trials for patients with rheumatoid arthritis. Also includes a personal notification service of new clinical trials.

CENTERWATCH
www.centerwatch.com
One of the more established sites around, CenterWatch is a comprehensive site with patient information and a notification service.

RHEUMATOLOGY RESEARCH INTERNATIONAL
www.rri.net

Books

Every month new books on arthritis are released. Originally, I ate them up like a hungry child. As I begin to better understand my arthritis needs, I began to be more exclusive about which books I read. Each of us has certain needs that take priority over others, and there is a book appropriate for every need. A good reference point is to seek books by people with experience (lots of experience) who have distinguished themselves among the arthritis and rheumatology professional communities. A good starting point is to check out the books published and endorsed by the Arthritis Foundation or other patient organizations at www.arthritis.org, or call (800) 283-7800.

When impacted by arthritis, it is easy to become too narrowly focused on disease-specific information. I discovered that some of the best coping and self-understanding came through books not specific to arthritis, but relevant to managing disease and coping. These are the ones I highly recommend.

Mending the Body, Mending the Mind by Joan Borysenko, Ph.D. Addison-Wesley Publishing: New York, 1993.

Getting Well Again by O. Carl Simonton, M.D., et al. Bantam Books: New York, 1992.

The Power of Positive Thinking by Rev. Norman Vincent Peale. Ballantine Books: New York, 1996.

When Bad Things Happen to Good People by Harold S. Kushner. New York, 1997.

Feel Good: The New Mood Therapy by David Burns, M.D. New York, 1999.

The Feeling Good Handbook by David Burns, M.D. Plume Books: New York, 1999.

Guidance on Arthritis and Related Topics

ACCESS TO MEDICATIONS

Today, management and control of arthritis relies heavily upon the appropriate use of medications. Anti-inflammatory, disease modifying, immuno-suppressive, and biologic medications can slow or halt the progression of inflammation and deformities. But many of these medications are expensive by anyone's budget. While nothing can take the place of having money or decent health insurance to pay for medications, there are some programs to assist if you have the appropriate qualifications. A good starting point is the American College of Rheumatology page on assistance programs at www.rheumatology.org/patients/assistance.htm.

Rx Assist
www.rxassist.org
Rx Assist, sponsored by Robert Wood Johnson Foundation, includes a list-

ing of the pharmaceutical manufacturers who offer pharmaceutical patient assistance programs. In all cases, the door to these programs is your physician.

MEDICARE
www.medicare.gov/prescription/home
While Medicare does not yet provide a prescription drug benefit, this site provides direction for prescription drug assistance programs run by individual states.

COMMUNICATION

It may be difficult to secure the help you feel you need when you have not resolved how arthritis impacts your daily life. Asking for help may seem difficult for some people, but it is not a sign of weakness. Learning what motivates you and how others perceive your words, and being specific about the help you need are key elements to getting help. A general book about communication, *The Dance of Connection: How to Talk to Someone When You're Mad, Hurt, Scared, Frustrated, Insulted, Betrayed or Desperate* by psychotherapist Harriet Lerner (2001), can be helpful.

COPING

While many websites provide information about arthritis, coping with the many facets of arthritis requires person-to-person contact and communication. Self-help and mutual-aid groups have proven effective in dispelling fear and myths and promoting a sense of well-being. Seek out support and self-help groups through patient organizations, online chat rooms, and medical institutions. Being alone in dealing with arthritis is not conducive to good emotional and physical health. Coping with arthritis is a family affair, so also seek out groups for spouses and siblings.

DEPRESSION

Depression is common among people with chronic diseases, so the first step is to realize that depression may be related to arthritis. Seeking professional help, support, and mutual-aid groups, and finding willing friends to whom you can communicate your feelings to develop a plan of action can help you see more clearly. Writing in a journal and talking into a tape recorder can also help you express your feelings. I cried into a tape recorder for days until I began to snicker with laughter about the situation in which I found myself. That ultimately led to writing down a checklist of things I could do to seek better medical and emotional care. Dr. David Burns's book *Feel Good: the New Mood Therapy* (1999) also helped me.

DISABILITY BENEFITS

If you cannot work because of arthritis or rheumatic disease, you may qualify for financial help from the federal or state government. This differs from country to country. Check with patient organizations and their websites for further information. A good starting point is the Arthritis Foundation at www.arthritis.org/Resources/disability__benefits.asp.

DISABILITY INSURANCE

If you have worked, you may qualify for long-term disability insurance offered through your employer or through an individual insurance plan. A good starting point is the U.S. Social Security Administration at www.ssa.gov/OP__Home/rulings/di-toc.html.

EMPLOYMENT/WORKPLACE

In the United States, we are fortunate enough to have the Americans with Disabilities Act (ADA) to assist us in the workplace. But working with the regulations, translating it appropriately with your employer, and building equality for your skills at work can still be daunting. Working with your immediate supervisor and human resources department, and understanding your rights in the context of the ADA are important. You may find that how you communicate your workplace needs may be just as important as knowing what your needs really are. As a former human resources manager, I found that communication style is vital to getting what you need in order to be considered equal among peers. Check out the ADA homepage at www.usdoj.gov/crt/ada/adahom1.htm.

EXERCISE

Maintaining an appropriate exercise regimen is vital to keeping fit and promoting muscle and joint health. Knowing what type of exercise is right for you given your arthritis-affected areas is the domain of a quality physical therapist. Once you establish a routine, you can move up to enhanced regimens. Start with a referral from your physician to an appropriate exercise-training facility with personnel who are knowledgeable about your limitations. Strength training used to be ill advised for people with arthritis, but recent research is now dispelling that myth. Educate yourself by checking the consumer information offered by the American Physical Therapy Association at www.apta.org/Consumer or the Arthritis Foundation at www.arthritis.org.

FINDING THE RIGHT DOCTOR

Physicians differ in their personalities and styles of practice, just as patients differ in their coping and arthritis-management styles. But finding the right physician to help you manage arthritis is critical to good health. I firmly believe that a person with mild to severe arthritis should been seen regularly by a rheumatologist. In some countries, an orthopaedic surgeon/rheumatologist is most appropriate for the person with arthritis. In other countries, primary-care physicians are the only ones in sufficient supply to handle the growing numbers of people with arthritis. Good starting points are the referral list of board-certified rheumatologists maintained by chapters of the Arthritis Foundation and talking with people whom you've met in support or mutual-aid groups who like their physician and speak well of their care.

GOAL SETTING

I learned that setting goals helped me to overcome the physical trauma and emotional setbacks imposed by arthritis. Each day and each week, I set small, manageable goals for myself, such as increasing the number of repetitions of an exercise or taking medications as directed. An important element to setting goals is finding appropriate incentives for jobs well done—the rewards of goal setting. For me, they included delicious pieces of salami, treating myself to a facial, or watching a favorite movie! Whatever your goals, be sure to attach them to incentives to move you to action and contentment. You might want to read *The Magic Lamp: Goal Setting for People Who Hate to Set Goals* by Keith Ellis (Three Rivers Press: New York, 1998).

HEALTH INSURANCE

Getting health insurance is difficult; working with it may be even more cumbersome. Employer-based group insurance is by far the most efficient way to secure insurance. The same may be true for self-employed individuals with arthritis who have at least two other employees. Many patient organizations offer patient-advocate volunteers or health professionals to assist in dealing with health insurance difficulties. Many health insurance companies now offer case managers to monitor and provide a central point of information about your case. Maintaining good records and keeping copies of each medical treatment invoice and a chart of what was paid by your health insurance will help you sleep better at night.

INSPIRATION/MOTIVATION

Finding your inner well of strength and motivation to get past the pain and emotional upset of arthritis can be fatiguing. Maintaining an appropriate exercise and range-of-motion movement program can be worse than staying on a diet. Where do you get that inner strength to keep at it? Some practice meditation, prayer, spirituality, or focusing. Some have a resolute belief that they are worth the multiple efforts of managing their arthritis. Others find energy in the support structure of family and friends. The key is to find what works for you. I continue to use a combination of all these methods, but mostly I have come to believe that I am a good and decent person of worth who has much to offer and much to give this universe. Working to keep myself healthy is a labor of love. You may want to check out books such as the Bible, *The Power of Positive Thinking* by Rev. Norman Vincent Peale (1996), *Success Through a Positive Mental Attitude* (1996), and *Think and Grow Rich* (2001) by Napoleon Hill.

MEDICATIONS

Knowledge about your arthritis medications and the class of medications that you take is important to managing arthritis and communicating with your physician, dentist, or other health professionals. Knowing about potential side effects and how to maximize your medications' effectiveness is also important. A good starting point is the Arthritis Foundation's Drug Guide at www.arthritis.org/conditions/DrugGuide/default.asp.

PAIN AND FATIGUE MANAGEMENT

Pain and fatigue management are inherent parts of living with any form of arthritis. Learning how to recognize when you have met your threshold for fatigue and pain are keys to maintaining an active lifestyle. Good starting points include the Arthritis Foundation at www.arthritis.org and the American Pain Foundation at www.painfoundation.org.

PARENTING

Parenting with arthritis or parenting a child with arthritis carries a host of strategic considerations. Education remains the key to devising a life that brings happiness from being a parent in special situations. An invaluable resource is the American Juvenile Arthritis Organization at www.arthritis.org/communities/children_young_adults.asp. My friends Earl Brewer, M.D., and Kathy Angel have also authored a great book: *Parenting a Child with Arthritis: A Practical Empathetic Guide to Help You and Your Child Live with Arthritis.* Other great books include the Arthritis Foundation's *Raising a Child with Arthritis: A Parent's Guide* (1998) and *Your Child with Arthritis: A Family Guide for Caregiving* by Lori Tucker, M.D., et al. (2000).

RELATIONSHIPS

Dating and maintaining significant-other relationships have continually been hot issues at young adult conferences. Unfortunately, there are no magical steps. But allowing your own personality to shine through arthritis, and developing hobbies, interests, and a zest for life are factors that attract people, as are self-confidence and a healthy sense of self-esteem. Finding your sense of inner beauty while learning to make the most of your external features is another plus. While as of yet there are no books that address this issue in arthritis (although I'm working on it!), just being able to talk to others in a similar situation through support and mutual-aid groups can prove fruitful. Check with your local patient organization.

SCHOOL AND COLLEGE

Dealing with arthritis in the school or college environment can be very challenging. Educating your teachers, principal, or professors can go a long way to getting the appropriate accommodations. Communicating your needs to your teacher and fellow students can help maintain your intellectual focus despite any physical challenges. A good starting point is the American Juvenile Arthritis Organization, a division of the Arthritis Foundation, which has produced a variety of information pamphlets to help in the school setting at www.arthritis.org/communities/children_young_ adults.asp.

SENSUALITY AND SEXUALITY

Having arthritis doesn't mean you stop being human. Expressing your sense of sensuality should be as important as brushing your teeth, but we sometimes minimize our sensuality and thus our sexuality because of arthritis pain, fatigue, and limitations in function. Understanding and acknowledging your sensual feelings and your human right to have these feelings is the first step. The Arthritis Research Campaign has a terrific information booklet available at www.arc.org.uk/about_arth/booklets/ 6037/6037.htm.

SPORTS

Enjoying sports despite having arthritis depends on the severity of your arthritis. Most can enjoy some sort of low-impact sport such as swimming, gardening, or even golf. Working with your physician is key to maintaining cardiovascular exercise without damaging precious bones and joints. Have an honest discussion with your physician. Also check out the free pamphlets from the Arthritis Foundation on a variety of sports at www.arthritis.org.

SELF-HELP DEVICES

Everyday devices and special ones made specifically for people with limited grip strength, grasp, or reach can be the difference between being independent or not. My home is filled with them. They all fall under "what a great idea" category for making life easier and more efficient. Mail-order catalogs are full of novel gadgets for the kitchen, office, bath, car, traveling, garden, outdoors, parenting, and sporting. Check out the Easy to Use products endorsed by the Arthritis Foundation, Ability Hub: Assistive Technology Solutions at www.abilityhub.com and mail-order catalogs.

SURGERY

Surgery still remains an option for people with arthritis when medications fail to halt or slow disease progression. After seventeen surgeries, I understand my role to ensure a joint-replacement success. Dealing with the emotional aspects of what to expect, how you are treated in the hospital, and post-operative rehabilitation are issues in which you have the strongest voice in how you handle, cope with, and survive any surgery. Good starting points are support and mutual-aid groups along with the Arthritis Foundation's Surgery Center at www.arthritis.org/conditions/SurgeryCenter/default.asp or the American Academy of Orthopaedic Surgeons patient information center at http://orthoinfo.aaos.org.

TRAVEL

Travel for fun or business with arthritis can be burdensome without appropriate planning. I log more than 100,000 miles each year in my work and I still love to travel. Simple strategies, such as making advance reservations, finding seats with enough legroom, and working with your airline to secure wheel chair assistance or baggage assistance, can make the difference between an arthritis flare or pure travel enjoyment. A good place to start is with my friend Carol Eustice's guide to arthritis at about.com at http://arthritis.about.com/cs/travel.

ADVOCACY

Such a little word can mean so much! I have found that being an advocate is my passion because it means sticking up for myself, my needs, and people like me. Becoming an advocate is as simple as sharing with others how arthritis affects your life, be it through a letter to the editor of your newspaper, or visiting your legislative representative, school principal, professor, employer, insurance company, or neighborhood store. It is stepping forward with the belief that in order to function in this society, certain laws, rules, or practices need to change to help you play on an equal playing field. It is vigorous education of those who do not know about arthritis. The Arthritis Foundation and the American College of Rheumatology are seeking patient advocates to help share the stories about arthritis with legislative decision-makers. Getting a grip on arthritis and living well with arthritis means becoming your strongest ally and advocate.

To contact Amye Leong for speaking engagements, email: bunderwood@penguinputnam.com or amye@healthymotivation.com.

way it worked for them, of course. Patients came into their lives, accepted their care, and moved on. Rarely, however, did anyone stay for ninety-three days. In fact, I left Daniel Freeman arthritis rehab as the official single-stay record holder (and the mark still stands today). For the staff, the job would go on. There would be new patients, but similar work. For me, life was about to change dramatically, and I felt more than a little anxious about it. Just before I left, I looked around the room one last time. I looked into the tiny closet, which held four items of clothing (all I ever needed). I looked in the bathroom. I looked down the hall. I took a deep breath and held it: *I want to remember what this room looks like. I want to remember what it smells like, sounds like. I want to feel it . . . taste it. Because I am never coming back here again!*

My discharge was based on the fact that I had reached a point of "physical stability," which was, after all, the stated goal of the program. But that hardly meant I had recovered. Stability, in my case, still meant being unable to walk. It meant being unable to eat in a restaurant without having people stare at me. It meant having hands and feet that were horribly deformed.

Along with my discharge papers I was given a set of at-home exercises. We're not talking Jane Fonda or Kathy Smith here, folks. We're talking about movements that most able-bodied people would not even consider exercise, like lying on your bed, pointing your toes to the sky, and holding the position for a count of ten. That was the extent of it. I was still in pretty bad shape. I had been dependent in the hospital, and the truth was, I would be dependent when I left the hospital. My mom and dad would have to help me with the simplest of tasks, like washing my hair, cutting my food, even going to the bathroom. It made me feel like a baby. At the same time, there was a level of comfort in knowing that I was going